**MORE FUN
THAN WE EVER
EXPECTED**

Proton Therapy for Prostate Cancer

**MORE FUN
THAN WE EVER
EXPECTED**

Proton Therapy for Prostate Cancer

**BILL & KAREN DEMBOSKI
MITCH & LOIS MCGUIRE**

Cover design by Elsa Holderness
Printed in the United States of America
Interior design by Serbin Printing, Inc. · Sarasota, Florida

ISBN 978-0-9824611-5-0

Library of Congress Control Number: 2010913639

Visit: protontherapyforcancer.com

10 9 8 7 6 5 4 3 2 1

First Edition

Contents

Acknowledgements

As the four authors of this book, we would like to thank the many patients and their wives whom we met at the University of Florida Proton Therapy Institute (UFPTI) in Jacksonville, Florida. Like us, they had a wonderful experience there, and they felt it was important to get the word out about this exceptional facility. They encouraged us to write this book about our experiences for the sake of all the men who have to deal with prostate cancer as well as their wives and other loved ones who become their caregivers and provide critical emotional support.

A special thanks to the entire staff at UFPTI for their support and professionalism. We never felt like patients or wives of patients, but always part of a special family. We often felt like we were on a cruise ship instead of dealing with cancer therapy.

This was due, in large part, to the efforts of Gary Barlow and Gerry Troy. They were supported by the Executive Director, Stuart Klein, and the Executive Medical Director, Dr. Nancy Mendenhall. These people have helped create an incredible culture of caring and respect.

After we started this book, Gerry Troy retired and Bradlee Robbert was promoted to Patient Services Department, replacing Gerry. We have met with Bradlee and can truly say they have promoted the right person to continue their high standards regarding the patient culture. Bradlee has been a registered radiation therapist since 2003 and has worked in photon, proton, brachytherapy, and electron therapy. He is using his clinical experience to help provide patients with a full understanding of their treatments, while creating a community of support between patients during their journey of fighting cancer.

The people you first meet are the friendliest, most caring and helpful people you will meet anywhere.

They all carried smiles and warm attitudes. Interaction with these people felt like a warm fuzzy blanket.

The therapists were professional, caring individuals, and they all had a great sense of humor.

Our special thanks go to all the test readers who found many mistakes and made so many good suggestions.

Finally, we'd like to thank the four proton patients, Bill Norrell, Gary Smith, Paul Preuss, and Dan Cibock, who contributed their personal stories regarding prostate cancer and UFPTI to this book.

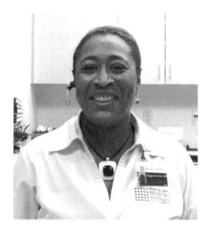

*From Maggie
at the nurses'
station, to*

*Roscoe, the
front door guard,*

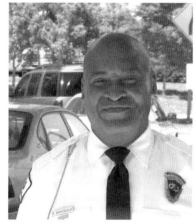

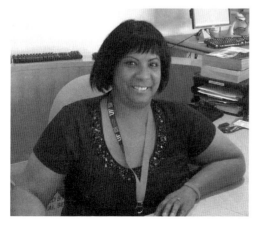

*and Dina at the
reception desk,
everyone was
wonderful*

Foreword

More *Fun than We Ever Expected* may seem like an odd subtitle for a book dealing with prostate cancer. After all, how much fun can prostate cancer be? One in 35 men will die of this disease. It's the second leading cause of cancer death in men after lung cancer. Nearly 200,000 men will be diagnosed with the disease this year.

For the two male authors of this book there certainly wasn't any fun in being diagnosed with this terrible disease. There wasn't much fun involved with researching and finding out the potential treatments and their possible side effects which include incontinence and sexual dysfunction.

After receiving the diagnosis of prostate cancer, there definitely wasn't much fun in dealing with some doctors. Unbelievably, many of them didn't even mention proton therapy as one of the options for treatment of prostate cancer.

Yet, the subtitle of this book is not just meant to be an attention getter. The authors' prostate cancer journey eventually led them to the University of Florida Proton Therapy Institute in Jacksonville, and it was there that they had ***more fun than they ever expected***. They received world class treatment in a world class facility by a world class group of people.

The treatment time each day was minimal and the side effects were mild or nonexistent. Because of that, patients were able to spend a large portion of their day playing golf, attending dinners, and enjoying other activities.

The authors' experiences were extremely positive, and they are determined to share those experiences with as many people as possible. They believe strongly that anyone who receives a prostate cancer diagnosis should consider proton therapy treatment. It has become their mission to tell as many people as possible about proton therapy. This book is part of that effort.

The authors intend to donate one third of any profits from this book to the University of Florida Proton Therapy Institute in Jacksonville, Florida (UFPTI). They hope that the money might help UFPTI continue to improve proton therapy for the treatment of prostate cancer.

Introduction to the Prostate
The Prostate

A normal-sized prostate fits neatly into the crowded, multi-functional area of the man's lower pelvis.

The prostate in men, like the breast in a woman, is a gland that produces and secretes fluid and controls the flow of fluid. Cells lining the prostate gland make some of the semen that comes out of the penis at the time of sexual climax (orgasm).

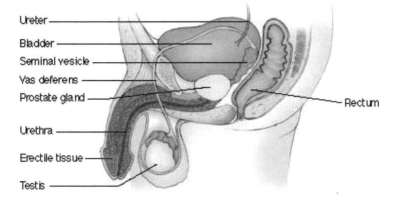

Prostate-specific antigen (PSA) helps to keep the semen in its liquid form. It is an enzyme in the form of a glycoprotein produced primarily by cells lining the acini and ducts of the prostate gland.

A normal human male prostate is about the size of a small plum. The prostate sits above the base of the penis below the urinary bladder and backs onto the front wall of the rectum.

The prostate evolved in this tight-wedged position to aid reproduction. The prostate makes some of the fluid for semen, may keep urine out of the semen, and enhances pleasurable sensations of arousal and orgasm.

In males a single pipe, the urethra, serves two functions, urination and ejaculation. The urethra runs from the bladder through the prostate to the tip of the penis. The section that runs through the prostate is called the prostatic urethra.

The prostate gland makes almost a third of the fluid in the semen that a man ejaculates.

During ejaculation millions of sperm arrive in the prostatic urethra. The sperm are made in the testicles.

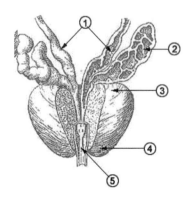

1: Vas deferens
2: Seminal vesicle
3: Base of the prostate
4: Apex of the prostate
5: Prostatic urethra

Leading from each testis is a coiled mass of spermatic ducting called the epididymis (Greek: upon + testicle), which houses maturing sperm. The epididymis, (below left), looks like the crest on a helmet. It connects to a tube called the vas deferens (Latin: carrying-away vessel).

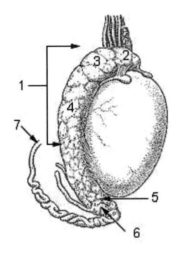

Sperm lodge in the epididymis for several days. When sexual excitement triggers ejaculation, muscle contractions in the wall of the vas deferens suck the sperm from the epididymis through to the vas deferens. As muscle contractions continue in waves the sperm rocket up towards and around the bladder and down by the two seminal vesicles into the prostatic urethra.

Some of the prostate is made of muscle. When sperm reach the prostatic urethra the prostate contracts, this may pinch a duct to the bladder so that sperm are kept urine-free. The contraction helps secrete prostatic fluid into the urethra and may also help expel the ejaculate.

CHAPTER 1

The Bill Demboski Story

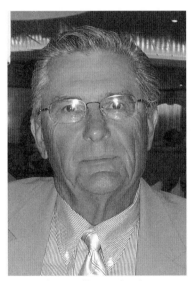

Coauthor Bill Demboski

B ill was 72 years old when diagnosed with prostate cancer. He is physically active and likes to golf, hunt, and fish. His goal as he researched the treatments for prostate cancer was to find a therapy that didn't drastically change his life.

I was having a routine physical examination in April of 2009, and I didn't expect the results to be any different than my last physical. I went to my doctor's office to get the results of all the tests he had ordered as part of my exam.

During his review, my doctor was alarmed at my high Prostate-Specific Antigen (PSA) Test. It had jumped from 6 to 8.3. His concern was the poor ratio between PSA and free PSA.

He suggested I see my urologist. I explained I had a scheduled appointment within three weeks and assured him I would keep the appointment. I didn't give the incident much thought after the review.

Back in 1994, when my doctor in Pennsylvania had performed a digital rectal examination (DRE) he felt a lump on one side of my prostate. That lump, along with my PSA of 4.5, prompted him to schedule a biopsy with a local urologist within two weeks. When I visited the urologist, he assured me the biopsy procedure was relatively painless and it would only take a few minutes.

Now, I won't say he lied, but there should be some law against severe distortion of the facts. The procedure was neither short nor painless. No pain medication was administered and the whole process reminded me of a torture exercise designed for World War II. In about an hour it was complete, after the doctor and his assistant managed to stuff a softball-sized instrument up my rectum and rip out six samples of tissue from my prostate.

The samples were sent to the laboratory for pathology studies. I must admit those ten days were a little trying, and I often had thoughts about the big IF. What would I do IF the results were positive? IF the results indicated cancer, what would the treatments be like?

I was anxious when I called the doctor's office and identified myself, requesting my results. The nurse said I needed to talk to the doctor but he was busy seeing patients. Would I call back?

This really got my mind working overtime in high gear. I told myself, "*It can't be good news or the nurse would have told me the results. This can't be happening to me. I have a life to live.*"

I called back in an hour and asked for the doctor. I was put on hold for about a minute before the doctor got on the phone. He didn't mince words. "You're fine. No cancer. Have a great life."

Great news! Of course, I had expected this result all along. Hell, I was bulletproof and something like cancer couldn't happen to *me*.

When I went to see my current urologist in May of 2009, I heard the concern in his voice about the *free PSA ratio*, a term that was unfamiliar to me. I asked him to explain his concerns about the ratio.

He said that along with total PSA, my primary doctor had ordered a free PSA. This ratio determines how much unbound PSA was in the bloodstream. The higher the free PSA, the lower the chances one has of having cancer in the prostate. He stated that my free PSA was very low and he recommended a prostate biopsy.

Immediately my mind rewound to 1994 and the barbaric process of harvesting tissue samples. Besides, the facts were that nothing was found. I also knew there was a lot of controversy regarding the number of false positives associated with this test. Naturally, being the *compliant* patient that I was, I said to my doctor, "There's no way in Hell I'm going through that again just to hear that I'm fine! Have a nice life!"

Thank God for some very caring doctors like mine. My doctor was very patient with my fears and explained how the process of biopsy had changed. I would be given general anesthesia and would have no pain or recollection of the procedure.

Well, OK then. No pain and no memory. I could handle that. I was scheduled for a biopsy in a few days.

The doctor didn't exaggerate. The biopsy was as the doctor had described and I had no pain or recollection of the procedure.

A week passed and my wife, Karen, and I sat in my urologist's office, waiting for the results. I was not too concerned since I was bulletproof. My thoughts returned to 1994 and the negative report. I was light and cheerful, expecting only the best.

The doctor walked in, sat down, and explained the biopsy report based on the 12 samples taken. He also showed us a prostate map indicating the locations from which the samples were drawn. "I have good news and bad news," he said.

With no break in his discussion, he said I had CANCER, but he said that it was caught early and it wasn't an aggressive form. The bottom line: I wasn't going to die from this and there were lots of treatment options available, options that weren't available ten years ago. He then discussed the therapy options and his recommendations.

At that point I didn't hear much more, as my mind reeled in disbelief. I was not supposed to get cancer! I was bulletproof!

I kept looking at my wife. She seemed pretty calm and accepted the news with stoic grace. My wife and I were both married before; I was divorced and she had lost her husband to heart disease following a 15-year ordeal. I looked for any signs of anguish or despair on her face. There were none.

After that, the doctor said something to me that I think is *critically* important:

You are ultimately responsible for your health and choice of therapy. All of the options have advantages and disadvantages, and you have to decide which is right for you and your wife. Talk to a lot of people who've survived prostate cancer. Learn all you can about each type of therapy. Remember, when you talk to doctors who perform a specific therapy, they will all tout their therapy as your best option. If all you have is a hammer, everything else looks like a nail.

Don't be taken in by one therapy because the facility is close to home or you like the doctor. Get on the Internet and research everything you can about prostate cancer therapy. Believe me, there is a lot to go through.

I would listen to my doctor's words intently and subsequently follow his advice during the research phase of my decision-making process.

Then my doctor said, "Don't be panicked into doing something. There is a lot of time and you will *not* die from this disease. You may die *with* prostate cancer, but chances are something else will end your life. Now, we can meet again in a month and discuss your questions at that time."

My wife and I left his office. I was stunned! We really didn't need this disruption in our life. I was retired in Florida, playing golf, painting, fishing, and I was enjoying many social activities with friends. Every year Karen and I took a long vacation to locations we both had dreamed of seeing all of our working lives.

I had heard a lot of horror stories about prostate cancer—about incontinence, bowel problems, and other unpleasant stuff. Was this what I had to look forward to? Was my great life over or about to be?

Thank God for the Internet! It is a great tool to gather information. Karen and I took my doctor's advice to heart and spent six to eight hours a day both searching and reading the information that we gathered.

It was during this phase that I discovered proton therapy, which had never been mentioned by my urologist. I began to study and gather information about other treatments including surgery (not recommended by my urologist), photon radiation, radiation seeds, cryogenics, ultrasonic, and thermal ablation.

The information began to accumulate. It was easy to

find the information and request additional details from the sources I discovered. However, it didn't take long to get overwhelmed with the massive amounts of data we were collecting.

As the material came in, I would do a quick sort and try to identify the most important portions of the information. After awhile, it started to all run together. Karen and I tried to keep organized with file folders. They helped us go back and retrieve data we might have missed, or find answers to questions we might have overlooked as we reviewed the literature.

After two weeks of gathering information, we spent another two weeks reading, studying, and analyzing the therapies available. Karen would read the material after me, and then we'd discuss some of our findings. We never committed to any therapy during that process. Our mission was only to gather and study the data.

After two weeks of study, we decided to determine what therapy we felt would be most appropriate for me and Karen. One factor we had to consider was my four bouts with ulcerative colitis which began in 1960. Anything we chose had to be gentle, causing little or no collateral damage. I didn't want to exchange cancer for chronic colon problems.

The following is the list we developed of potential treatment options, which includes a brief summary of our conclusions about each one:

Types of Therapy Available

Surgery: Not recommended due to many side effects; e.g. urinary incontinence and erectile dysfunction. Greatly affects the quality of life and has a long convalescing time. Secondary infection is highly probable.

Radiation: There are two types of radiation currently used to treat cancer: (1) Photon Radiation, (also known as X-ray radiation) is commonly accepted in place of surgery. We heard many stories of bad side effects after treatment. When the radiation exits the target site, it destroys healthy cells. Also, X-ray radiation is a known cancer producer and secondary cancer is possible. An advantage of X- ray radiation is that it usually can be performed locally and no one needs to know you are in cancer therapy, if that is important to you. (2) Proton radiation is also used to kill cancer cells but is a completely different modality and does not produce exit energy and is not known to cause secondary cancer when used.

Cryogenic Ablation: Not recommended by my doctor. Freezing parts of the prostate kills cancer cells, but has a high probability of sexual dysfunction.

Brachytherapy: While gaining popularity with patients, there are unsolved technical problems with seed radiation. The seeds are inserted into the prostate, but are known to migrate. They have been found in lungs, heart, bladder, and other body parts. Research is underway to make the seeds smaller and have them linked in a chain so as to minimize migration. After researching this therapy, we did not feel comfortable with this option. I didn't want radiation in my body capable of producing free radicals, which are known to cause cancer.

Watchful Waiting: Not recommended by the doctor. Because of my relative good health, active lifestyle, and youthful outlook and appearance (even though I was 72 years of age), I saw myself as too young to consider this option.

Thermal Ablation: Not recommended by the doctor. High temperatures are known to kill cancer cells. Using an infrared generator and heating the prostate causes cancer cells to die, but can affect healthy cells. Side effects include the risk of sexual dysfunction.

Proton Radiation Therapy: Scientists discovered that a proton particle will travel to a precise depth and give up most of its energy in a large burst when it reaches a predictable depth. Most of the energy is delivered to the target area. This process is called the Bragg Peak. The advantage is that there is minimal exit energy to cause damage to healthy tissue.

About a month after learning that I had prostate cancer, Karen and I were back in the urologist's office to discuss my choice of therapies. It turned out to be a great meeting.

When I informed Dr. W of our choice, he made no attempt to discourage or belittle proton therapy. In this regard, I was more fortunate than other patients I'd read about who had chosen proton therapy. In fact, Dr. W said that it was a good choice for me, even though he'd never mentioned proton therapy as an option during our previous visit.

He then asked me if I would like to talk to a former prostate cancer patient who had the *proton experience* at The University of Florida Proton Therapy Institute in Jacksonville, Florida. That man was currently cancer free. I accepted and Dr. W said he would contact the patient and have him call me. The man had requested confidentiality.

The next day I spent an hour talking to the man on the phone. I asked him about every aspect of his treatment experience, including any side effects. He had nothing but good things to say about the Proton Center and the therapy he'd received there. He had experienced no side effects of any kind.

I was extremely grateful for how quickly the man had contacted me and the time he'd spent with me on the phone. It made me thankful for the many helpful, caring people in this world.

The next day I spent a lot of time thinking about what message, if any, I should send to important people in my life. I considered myself to be very lucky to have had my cancer detected early. I wanted all my friends to be aware of how important the PSA test is, and while it has some false positives, it is the only test men have to detect prostate cancer. I also wanted to make all the men aware of the free PSA test and its role in giving another definitive dimension to prostate cancer testing.

I wanted to share my story and information so others would know about the therapy options. With that decision, I sent an e-mail to warn and inform everyone I knew, especially my family members. I believe it was a good decision. After that e-mail, a number of surviving prostate cancer patients contacted me and told me their stories, including the type of therapy they had chosen.

Not all stories were success stories, and some included tales of some pretty serious side effects. This only added to the information I was collecting. By this time, I felt comfortable discussing my situation with anyone and everyone.

The next step was to contact The University of Florida Proton Therapy Institute in Jacksonville and get some information and, hopefully, start the paperwork. At this point I was elated. No surgery or photon (X-ray) radiation for me, and everyone said their experience with proton therapy had been pain free, with few or no permanent negative side effects.

I contacted the Patient Intake Department and asked what I needed to do. They asked for some personal information and sent an overnight package to me. The package included information about their facility and some forms I needed to complete. I promptly filled out the forms that day and faxed them back to the patient coordinator.

I was psyched. I finally had a handle on proton therapy and the plan for treatment. Things were going my way.

Whoopee!

Everyone I had talked to said that the actual treatment time in the Proton Institute was less than one hour a day, so most patients had lots of time for sightseeing, playing golf, fishing, shopping, and other things. I was looking forward to going to Jacksonville and getting rid of this *cancer thing*.

At approximately 4:00 p.m. the following day, I got awful news. The patient coordinator called and said I had been rejected as a candidate by the Proton Center! That was the second biggest jolt I had received throughout this entire episode.

Why was I rejected? The patient coordinator explained that I had indicated that I'd had four bouts of ulcerative colitis, and one of the doctors would not sign off on my admission due to that fact.

I was stunned! Rejected? It didn't make any sense. I was looking for the most benign therapy and I was sure proton was the best in my case. Why should I choose standard X-ray radiation, which was known to cause colon problems?

At that point, I truly panicked. I was determined to have proton therapy. If I could not be treated in Jacksonville, which was convenient and close to my home in Sarasota, I would go to Loma Linda, California, or the University of Pennsylvania. I'd go to Massachusetts General or even wait until August and go to Oklahoma's new center which was just about ready to open.

Why would a doctor reject me? At this point, I was mad, upset, and angry. I stewed for awhile and had a few tirades to make myself feel better.

At that point, Karen reminded me of the contact with the proton patient my urologist had arranged, who had helped me so much. I checked my notes. He had given me the personal cell phone number of the doctor at the Proton Center in Jacksonville who had cared for him, Dr. Bill Mendenhall. The patient had spoken of Dr. Mendenhall with great affection, and he had told me it was OK to call Dr. Mendenhall anytime.

Before I called the doctor, I set up an appointment with my gastroenterologist and asked him if he would write a letter recommending proton therapy as the correct treatment for a patient with prostate cancer and ulcerative colitis. The letter was a thing of beauty and was very sincere, requesting my acceptance to the Proton Center in Jacksonville.

I then called Dr. Bill Mendenhall as suggested by my patient contact, and told him about my tale of rejection. He immediately said that I shouldn't worry. He would take me on as a patient and his assistant would be in touch with me soon. I faxed him the letter written by my gastroenterologist concerning my ulcerative colitis, and also sent a copy to the patient coordinator's office.

Within 12 hours, I was contacted by Dr. Mendenhall's assistant and an appointment was set up for my first consult visit and examination. This whole incident showed me the power of networking and talking to as many people as possible. I thank God for the patient friend with whom I had networked which had led to the contact with Dr. Mendenhall.

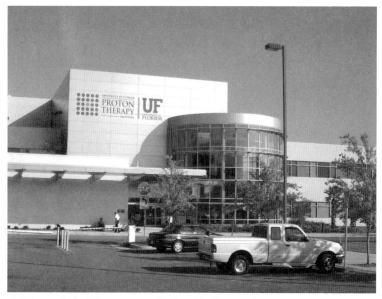

A View of the University of Florida Proton Institute, Jacksonville, Florida.

The Therapy Process: First Visit

The trip to Jacksonville from Sarasota was five hours and covered 250 miles. There were two main purposes for this visit: for me, to make sure I wanted to proceed with proton therapy; for the medical staff, to evaluate my health to ensure I was a good candidate for the therapy.

There was blood drawn for lab studies and a visit with the nurse. A general checkup was performed.

Proton therapy was in demand, and if my health was poor and my life span was at risk, the staff wouldn't proceed. I fully understood this situation. Fortunately, I passed their screening with no problems and was scheduled for a three-day visit. This visit would involve having a CT scan and MRI. Also, gold markers would be inserted into the prostate gland to make sure the targeted location received the proton radiation.

The Second Visit

Ten days later, we were on the way to Jacksonville again. We stayed at a local hotel that offered suites. During our stay there, we thought that hotel might be a good place to stay during the entire two months of the proton therapy treatments in the future.

As part of the three-day consult, we met with Dr. Mendenhall, who was to be my primary care physician while I was undergoing treatment. We discussed my situation and developed an understanding of expectations for myself, my wife, and my doctor.

One of my requirements was to keep my weight stable (plus or minus five pounds). I didn't think this would be a problem for me since I worked out and played golf one or two times a week. At that time, I didn't know how many parties, restaurants, and happy hours we would participate in with all the other patients and their wives that we were going to meet. Keeping a stable weight would be more of a challenge than I expected.

The consult also included more X-rays, CT Scans, and blood work. The last procedure was inserting the gold markers into the prostate, something I was dreading.

The procedure was not what I had anticipated. It was completed in a short time, with no pain. The doctor was very gentle in performing the insertion.

On the last day of the three-day consult, there was a tour of the facility. Gerry Troy gave us an excellent, informative tour, which gave us a clear idea of what was to come.

During our tour we met Mitch McGuire and his wife, Lois, from New Jersey, and we became instant friends. During our treatment time in Jacksonville, we were together for shopping, dinners, and exploring the area. We had a great time together, and we know we will remain friends always. Our relationship will be discussed more fully in chapters two and three.

The University of Florida Proton Therapy Institute said they would call within three days with a treatment schedule. After we returned to Sarasota, Florida, we received the call the next day informing us that my treatments would start on September 8. There will be much more detail about my actual treatment in Chapter 5.

Bill's Six-Month Checkup
By Karen Demboski

It had been six months and it was time for Bill's checkup in Jacksonville. I wondered what it would be like walking back into the Institute again. Would everyone still be warm and friendly?

I'm happy to say nothing had changed. Dina at the front desk actually recognized us. Doctor Bill and his nurse, Gail, were both as caring as ever.

Doctor Bill and Gail also had some great news. Bill's PSA was low! I was thrilled, to say the least.

Bill and I were in the mood to celebrate with great food and ice cream at City Kidz. Off we went for lunch. As soon as we walked into City Kidz, the owners, Clinton and Sonya, recognized us immediately. There were plenty of hugs and handshakes.

City Kidz had grown and it was very busy. After a great meal, we left feeling as full as ever. Bill and I promised Clinton and Sonya we'd stop back after our next medical visit.

It was rather nostalgic seeing the Third and Main complex again. Many fond memories of our two-month stay came back to us. We noticed that the neighborhood renovation was really coming along nicely with new businesses being established.

In this fast changing world, it was nice to see some good things still remain the same.

CHAPTER 2

The Mitchell McGuire Story

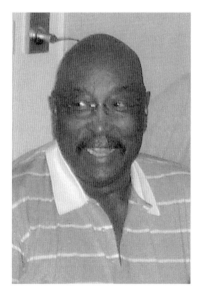

Coauthor Mitchell G. McGuire, Jr.

Mitchell McGuire was diagnosed with prostate cancer at the age of 66. He was looking for a treatment that didn't change his busy and active lifestyle or interfere with all his business activities.

I went for my annual physical in June of 2009 and, of course, got the usual tests. I expected the usual results, except the doctor gave me a digital rectal exam (DRE) this time. Upon examination, he said that my prostate seemed a little too firm and he referred me to a urologist. The urologist ordered a biopsy and this is where my story begins.

My wife, Lois, and I were sitting in the doctor's office waiting for our consultation and neither of us spoke very much. When the doctor entered the room and began to speak, all I heard was the word CANCER and I went blank. Thank God, Lois was there with me. Otherwise, I would not have been aware of anything else the doctor said after he uttered that word.

After the initial visit, I began to do some research while waiting for further testing. I had several friends who had been through this. One in particular had gone to Loma Linda, California, for proton therapy over ten years ago, and he highly recommended the treatment. I always remembered how happy he seemed throughout his treatment and how well he did after it was completed.

Proton therapy, in my mind, had so many advantages that I actually had suggested to another friend that he look into it when he informed me that he had prostate cancer. That was more than five years ago, and he is alive and well, presently living in the Sarasota area.

That same friend informed me that I didn't have to go to Loma Linda for proton therapy because they were presently offering the therapy in Jacksonville, Florida. He immediately gave me the phone number of Gerry Troy, the administrator of patient services, who had actually come to Jacksonville from Loma Linda.

I called Gerry and he immediately had a packet of information sent to me. It was in my hands within 24 hours. It included admission sheets and a requested history of my health.

Upon our arrival in Jacksonville for consultation in July, we went directly to Third and Main. A friend from the Jacksonville area had given us information about the facility. It was a brand new, gated, two-story apartment building with an elevator. The one and two bedroom apartments were completely furnished, with a TV in the bedroom and living room, telephone service, washer-dryer, a fully equipped kitchen, and all the linens you needed.

Because we lived so far from Jacksonville, the Proton Institute allowed us to do our one day visit on Friday, and our three day visit beginning the following Monday. The visit was fantastic! The staff at the Proton Institute was nothing less than wonderful! They were warm, friendly, positive, well-informed, and obviously very smart. They were able to answer any and all of our questions and put us at ease.

During our tour of the facility, I noticed that my wife and another pretty lady in the group kept talking, laughing, and seemed to be bonding as we went on the tour. This was really interesting, because normally that would not be my wife's *modus operandi*. The lady turned out to be Karen Demboski, whose husband, Bill, was a real hoot.

After the tour, we had a wine and cheese party right at the Proton Institute, who sponsored the event. Karen,

Bill, Lois, and I had a really fun time and Bill said, "We're supposed to be here for cancer treatment, and here we are—partying, drinking, and having a ball. Does that seem right? It feels like we're on a cruise!"

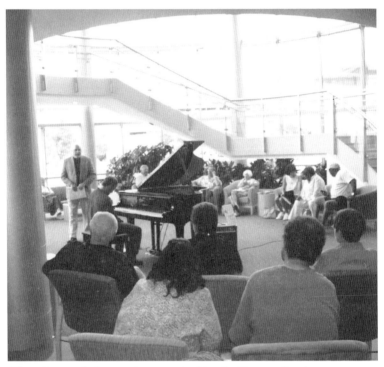

The wine and cheese piano recital in the Proton Institute

The wives exchanged numbers and thus began what we are sure will be a lifelong friendship. By the end of our three days, we were convinced that this was the place for proton therapy.

We were also convinced that Third and Main would be our home away from home while undergoing proton therapy. AJ, the building manager, was absolutely great. He did all he could to make our stay comfortable. He was pleasant, friendly, resourceful, and truly an asset to the facility. We made our reservations for our return visit and we were good to go.

My treatment began on August 26, 2009. When I first entered the University of Florida Proton Therapy Institute, I was greeted by a really wonderful lady named Kristy, who was my nurse. I had previously met her when I came for my intake and three-day workshop, but it was good to see her friendly face again, knowing she was thoroughly familiar with my case history.

I had expressed an interest in trying the shorter version of the treatment which consisted of 29 treatments instead of the traditional 39. Upon my return to begin treatment, Kristy advised Lois and me that I had been approved for the shorter version of the treatment. It consisted of the same amount of protons, but it provided a higher dose delivered over a shorter time. I was thrilled with the prospect because I would not have to be away from home and business in New Jersey for long. I was comfortable with our decision to go through the shorter version because I had every confidence in Dr. Henderson, my doctor throughout this journey.

I had already made up my mind that however long it took, I wasn't going to worry about anything during my time in Jacksonville. On the first day of treatment, however, I had some anxiety. Needless to say, Lois had just as much.

I wanted to make her feel at ease so I asked if she could accompany me into the treatment area. The therapists were super. They allowed my wife to come in with me. Once in there, they explained the process to both of us.

We ran into George Dollson, another newbie, in the lobby that morning. We had met him and his wife, Pat, on our three day visit. He said, "Mitch, it's a piece of cake. It doesn't hurt and you are in and out really fast."

He already had five treatments under his belt. He had been working out at the gym and had shot some pool that day, enjoying the good life.

George was so right. I was in and out in a flash and all the anxiety disappeared.

Within a week, the Demboskis arrived. Bill liked to play golf and that is my passion. Karen likes to shop and Lois puts the "S" in shop. I am certain the wives went to every mall in and around Jacksonville at least three times. I was glad that Lois had such a good friend in Karen living nearby.

The Demboskis, Lois, and I spent a lot of time together, mostly in the evening for dinner and/or cocktails. Karen makes delicious eggplant parmesan and Bill makes a mean martini. Sometimes we ate in, but most of the time we traveled around Jacksonville, checking out every kind of restaurant.

Make no mistake; it is difficult to be away from family and friends for such a long time. With that in mind, we took a two bedroom apartment at Third and Main in case we had visitors. We didn't have much time to ponder and worry about seeing our loved ones and friends.

Third and Main has a number of commercial enterprises on the first floor that are available to the public and are a convenience for the patients staying at the facility. One of the businesses established at Third and Main was an ice cream/sandwich store called City Kidz, with fantastic food and delightful owners.

In early September, our son, daughter-in-law, and our twin granddaughters came to visit. They were very excited and just loved going down to City Kidz each day for their favorite ice cream. Clint and Sonia, the proprietors, welcomed the girls, put on videos, and made them feel like family. The twins still speak of the ice cream parlor they visited when *Poppy* got his treatment. They don't actually know what *the treatment* was, but they sure enjoyed being there.

Two weeks later, our daughter, son-in-law, and 18-month-old grandson came to visit. We had a good time sightseeing and especially enjoyed visiting the Jacksonville Zoo. I had no interest in visiting a zoo and going on a train ride through it, but the things we do for love. To my surprise, it turned out to be a great experience. The Jacksonville Zoo was home to one of the largest gorillas I've ever seen.

A few days after the children left, Don and Gwen came to visit. They live in the Sarasota area and we have known them for years.

Don had had proton therapy more than five years earlier in Loma Linda, where he'd met Gerry Troy. He was aware of this *new* proton site in Jacksonville and had referred me to Gerry.

Don and I played golf with Bill almost every day while our caregivers, Gwen, Karen, and Lois, did what they like to do best—shop, get manicures and pedicures, wine and dine! We men always made it back for the wine part.

Several times we wanted to play golf and our treatment times got in the way of our tee times. Don't worry. The day that happened, Lois told me, "Now Boo Boo! Don't get confused. Get your priorities straight. You are here for prostate cancer treatment—not golf. Golf is just a fringe benefit."

Shortly after Don and Gwen's visit, we had a visit from our friends, Julius and Carla. They live half the year in Sarasota and half the year in Franklin Lakes, New Jersey. This was not just a pleasure visit. Julius had been diagnosed with prostate cancer, and he was there for a preliminary look at the Proton Institute.

We introduced Julius and Carla to Karen and Bill and everyone else we could. We were all so impressed with the care, concern, friendliness, and professionalism of the patients, doctors, and staff at the Institute.

Julius, being an engineer, was detail oriented, and he had dozens of questions for which he sought answers. When all was said and done, he became a patient of the Proton Institute in Jacksonville, Florida.

Carla fit right in and became a member of the Shopping and Beauty Treatment Club. Naturally, we all did our usual recreational activities and had a lot of fun.

I have so many fond memories of the parties on the breezeway at Third and Main. We would all bring a dish and some wine. Everyone was genuinely friendly and helpful.

As I went through my 29 treatments, I kept waiting for something to happen different or to go wrong, but it never did. I had no issues, no pain. I couldn't believe it! The biggest issue I had was once or twice I went through a period that I had a strong urge to urinate, especially during the night. Dr. Henderson advised me to take Advil each day. Bingo! That problem went away.

I exercised, lost a few pounds, my golf game improved, and my love life flourished. *Nothing* changed.

In the beginning of this process, I did an inordinate amount of research: books, doctors, the web, and many people who had been through some procedure for prostate cancer. I was consumed with the process, and why not? All that was at stake was my life!

After all was said and done, and when presented with all the options, I decided on proton therapy. Today, I am still sure it was the best decision I could have made. Through the entire process, from biopsy results to the last day of treatment, Lois and I maintained our strong faith in God and each other. Without that and the strong bond with our friends, the road we traveled would not have been as easy and as pleasurable. It was amazing how the time flew by.

When I completed my treatment, I was almost sorry to leave. Yes, I wanted to go back home to New Jersey, but I had also grown accustomed to having all the free time. It was great—golfing at will, dinner parties, cocktail hours, sleeping late, and just hanging out with friends.

Our last evening at Third and Main was spent with Bill and Karen, laughing, talking, sharing, and just having a good time. This was *Mitch's graduation* and we needed to make it special. Karen cooked eggplant parmesan with all the trimmings. We had a great time and we all had a ball just talking about our experiences.

We met for brunch the next morning at Cracker Barrel for our last goodbyes. None of us could help but feel a little sadness as Bill and Karen went back to Third and Main, and Lois and I soon headed north on Interstate 95 to New Jersey. However, there was also great joy that the cancer treatments we were so afraid of turned out to be the source for more fun than we could have ever imagined. This was largely due to the camaraderie and all the great people who we met, who were going through the same treatment.

Mitchell's Six-Month Check-up
Lois McGuire

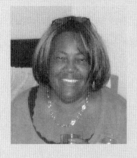

Wife to Mitchell and business partner, Lois was most concerned about getting her husband and partner back after going through whatever treatment was chosen.

It had been six months since Mitchell completed his proton treatments and he was doing well. It was time for Mitchell and me to return to Jacksonville for his six month checkup.

The day before our trip, I couldn't help thinking back to six months earlier. Finding out Mitchell had prostate cancer had been an experience I'd never forget. It was so very scary and I felt as if a rug had been pulled out from under me.

Mitchell had gotten an annual physical every year for more than 30 years so how could this have happened? How could he have a medium-grade cancer when last year they saw nothing?

Back then, when we arrived in Jacksonville for Mitchell's preliminary screening, I was numb. After our meeting with his case nurse, Kristy, and then Dr. Henderson, I began to feel so much better. Their knowledge and skill were so apparent. The more we talked with them, the more confidence we gained. They were so very kind. I knew by the end of the interview that this was the right treatment for us. If Mitchell was determined to be a good candidate for proton therapy, this was the treatment for him. Later, we both felt relieved when they determined Mitchell was a good candidate.

Once we returned to Jacksonville several weeks later, It didn't take us long to become familiar with the program, the people, our living space at Third and Main, and the wonderful people we met who made our stay so easy and so much fun.

We rented a two bedroom apartment at Third and Main and it was nice and homey. We took two bedrooms so that our children and their families could visit and be comfortable. The apartment came completely furnished with everything one could need to make living there a pleasant experience, and pleasant it was.

A typical day for me was to wake up at whatever time I wanted, have breakfast with friends, go shopping, get a manicure/pedicure, get my hair done, have a wonderful lunch, shop some more, socialize with friends or read a novel, have cocktails, go to dinner with friends, have some more fun, got to bed, then start over in the morning! I often thought, "*It doesn't get any better than this.*"

I soon realized that I could be away from home and business and life would still go on. Mitchell and I had an opportunity to really get to know each other in a way that we couldn't when we were going to work every day, and dealing with life's issues and problems. We relearned how to rely on each other for company, support, fun, and all the other things that brought us together originally.

As I continued thinking about returning to Jacksonville the next day, it seemed a little odd that we were both excited to return. We were actually looking forward to a positive six month checkup at the Proton Institute. After that, we were eager to see and visit with several of our proton buddies who would also be returning for their six month checkups. We had even made arrangements to stay a few extra days to visit together and, of course, have some more fun.

The return visit to the Proton Institute lived up to our expectations. First and foremost, Mitchell's PSA was down to 1.6 and everything was going well. Again, the staff at the Institute helped make it a pleasure to be there.

We learned that Gerry Troy, a mainstay at the Institute, was retiring. As a matter of fact, it was his last day.

We were all sorry to see him leave because his patient services program was what got us through this difficult time and the many days of proton therapy. He will be missed, but the good news is, his legacy will linger on and his program has become an institution.

We attended the Wednesday luncheon which was kind of a farewell to Gerry as well as a testament to his fine work in promoting a positive experience for his patients. This luncheon happened each and every Wednesday and was open to proton patients and their guests. It was always extremely well organized, inspirational, and informative. The food was good too!

Again and again, I saw patients and former patients who had fond memories of their treatment, along with the fun they'd had with other patients. A main person responsible for the Wednesday luncheon was Dr. Henderson's mom, known affectionately as *Proton Mom*. She was lovely, warm, gracious, and caring. To have one of the doctor's moms be so involved and committed to service and to his work was more than impressive, it was a true blessing.

For me, one of the most impressive things about the staff and program at the University of Florida Proton Institute was the fact that the treatment was unique to the individual. Of all the patients in treatment for prostate cancer, a staggering number, each was treated on a person by person basis. This was not a cookie cutter approach.

On this trip to Jacksonville, we decided to stay at the Marriot Airport Residence Inn which was not more than five minutes from the Jacksonville Airport. This was where friends Julius and Carla were staying during Julius' treatment at the Proton Institute and they recommended it highly.

What a treat it turned out to be! The facility was very

nice with all the conveniences and a warm and friendly staff that make you glad you'd chosen to stay there. The facility provided a full breakfast and a happy hour, with hot food, beer, and wine for its guests each weekday. They also offered a special rate for long-term proton patients. The entire staff seemed genuinely invested in its guests having an enjoyable day. Additionally, hot tub, pool, and exercise rooms were available.

We found ourselves heading back to the Marriot Residence Inn each day for the five thirty happy hour, not necessarily for the food and drink, but for the conversation. Again, I thought to myself, "*We're here for a prostate cancer checkup, yet we're having such a positive social experience.*"

We arranged to meet other proton friends George and Pat Dollson in Jacksonville. George and Mitchell had scheduled their six month checkups to be at the same time. Along with Julius and Carla, we all had an absolute blast together each day with all the support of nice people who had a common bond.

It's not often that illness and adversity can have such a positive ingredient and outcome but this did and I remain excited and grateful to the University of Florida Proton Institute.

CHAPTER 3

Third and Main: A Wife's View

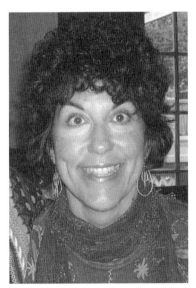

Karen, married to Bill Demboski, likes to travel and explore the world. During the initial diagnosis she spent an inordinate amount of time researching what therapy would be best suited for both her and her husband's lifestyle.

Coauthor Karen Demboski

Everything was going smoothly with Bill's work-up. This left one main issue—where were we going to live for two months? We were staying at a hotel. Although it had a separate bedroom, a fridge, and a microwave, it was far from being a *home* for two months.

Once a month, there's a piano concert at the Proton Institute performed by a local talent. While we were sipping wine at that event with Mitch and Lois McGuire, they asked us where we were going to stay while Bill was in treatment. We said we weren't sure, and they strongly suggested Third and Main. They were staying there for Mitch's work-up and intended to come back there during his treatment time. They gave us the phone number of AJ, the property manager. We immediately called AJ and set up an appointment for that afternoon to check it out.

Third and Main is an extended stay residence designed to be used specifically by proton patients. It has 36 residences with a gated entry, plenty of parking, and two restaurants on the first level. It's located ten blocks from downtown and five minutes from the Proton Institute.

When we arrived at Third and Main, we noticed it was located in Historic Springfield, an area that was going through a complete renovation. Although the streets and homes were undergoing lots of construction, it was clear this area was well on its way to becoming the wonderful neighborhood it had once been.

When we knocked on AJ's door, he immediately opened it, extended his hand, and displayed a huge smile. My first thought was *"How is a 17-year-old going to handle our needs?"*

The truth quickly became apparent. AJ was much older than 17. He just looked so young or maybe we were just getting older. Whatever the case, it soon became obvious AJ was extremely competent. He gave a great tour of the different apartment designs available and answered all our questions. The most important was, "What was the monthly rate for the apartment? At that time we were quoted $1450 per month, which included a balcony and we thought that was very reasonable. We knew immediately that this would be home for our two months in Jacksonville.

Through our entire time at Third and Main, AJ was great. If there was a problem, concern, or question, he took care of it quickly and efficiently. Most importantly, he was very kind. It was obvious he thought of us as family. He wanted everyone's treatment to go smoothly and our time there to be enjoyable.

A few weeks later we arrived there with all our stuff and began to get settled in our apartment. Mitch and Lois were first to greet us with a bottle of wine. We opened it and toasted the men and their treatment. Mitch had actually already started his a week earlier, and things were going very well for him.

We immediately started talking about all the great restaurants and stores they had checked out. However, the most important question was, "When and where were Mitch and Bill going to play golf?"

From that time forward, time just flew by. Lois and I became the shopping queens of Third and Main. Bill and Mitch golfed to their heart's content.

We met so many wonderful people at Third and Main. From the impromptu cocktail parties on the breezeway, to our group dinners at many local restaurants, to our going away get-together for Mitch and Lois, it was clear we had truly become a family. We all shared a common purpose—

to help get our men well. What a wonderful bond!

And while we're on the subject of food, drink, and good times, let me mention the two fabulous restaurants at Third and Main. City Kidz, a sandwich and ice cream shop, had the most wonderful crab cakes and chicken salad *ever.*

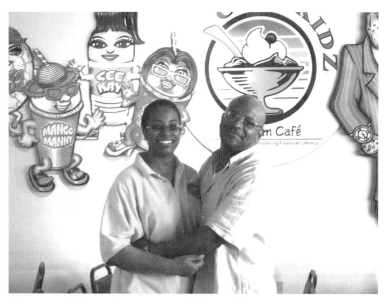

Sonya and Clint, Proprietors of City Kidz

You could top it off with great ice cream. Clint and Sonya, the proprietors, need to be thanked for some of our extra pounds and their *always* friendly support.

The second restaurant/deli is the Uptown Market. They serve a great take home dinner for two at a very reasonable price. This was wonderful, considering anyone that knows me, knows I hate to cook. Our best wishes to both restaurants for their continued success.

In closing, I have to admit I had some concerns about apartment living before moving to Third and Main. It had been years since I had to live in one, and I had always felt isolated when I'd lived in apartments before. There really seemed to be no such thing as neighbors. In the past, it seemed everyone was always too busy doing their own thing and had no time to get to know anyone else.

That certainly wasn't the case at Third and Main. The residents all had one thing in common, and the rest came naturally. The feelings of friendship and concern for everyone really made it a pleasant, comfortable home for everyone. The atmosphere was more like a college dorm than cold, apartment living.

Most importantly, no one ever felt alone or isolated and that's an important aspect of therapy. The cocktail parties gave our men a chance to discuss their knowledge and experiences, plus get answers to some of their questions in an atmosphere of concern and understanding. It truly was a big family away from home.

One of the perks offered by the Proton Institute was the membership they negotiated with the University Club. While you were a patient at the Institute, you were an automatic member of the Club with full member privileges. The normal initial fee is $1000 to join along with monthly dues of $100-$275. As a guest member it costs you "nothing" and you were only asked to follow the rules. The Club was located on the twenty-seventh floor of the Wachovia Building. It provided an unbelievable view of the town and the beautiful Florida sunsets.

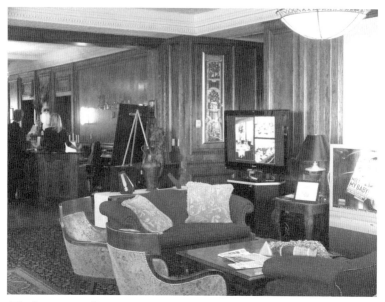

The lounge at the University Club

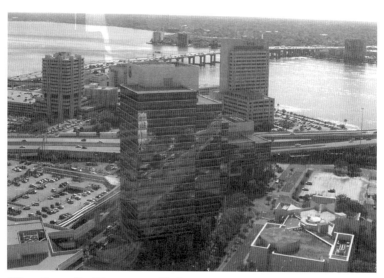

View from the University Club

They offered a great happy hour where good wines were just two dollars a glass. They also offered delicious finger food. Dinner was available in the bar area or in the dining room, with a jacket being required in the dining room. We held many graduation ceremonies at the University Club and toasted the graduates often. Bill and I both felt we had a much easier time with treatment because of the wonderful friendships we developed at the University Club.

A Special Visit from Special Friends

As Mitch and Lois stated, "When you're in need, your friends are there for you." Such was the case with Stan and Greta, a very dear couple who we look upon as our *family in Florida*.

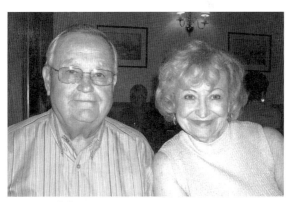

Stan and Greta

When they heard Bill and I were going to be in Jacksonville for two months, Stan and Greta immediately scheduled a support visit. They stayed at Third and Main, two apartments from ours, so logistics were no problem. We introduced them to all our new friends, went to dinner often, and visited all the shopping areas in Jacksonville. Bill and I could never thank them enough for all the support and the caring they showed during that time. As Mitch and Lois said, "True friends are a true blessing"—and we have been blessed.

The following are pictures of the good times at Third and Main that were mentioned earlier.

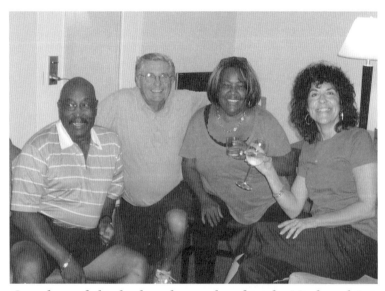

Coauthors of this book and now close friends, Mitch and Lois McGuire are from New Jersey. Mitch was Bill's golfing partner and Lois and Karen shopped their way around the Jacksonville, Florida, area. They enjoyed many dinners and wine together. All of this made the whole treatment experience very enjoyable.

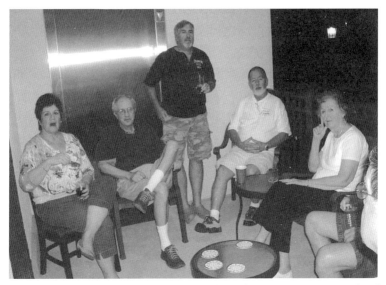

These were some of the patients that shared our experience at Third and Main while being treated at the Proton Institute.

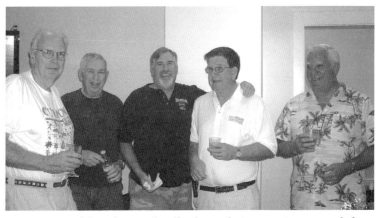

Patients would gather and talk about their experiences and share information. Sometimes we would just get together on the landings and everyone would bring something- food, wine or beer- and we would sit around and talk and get to know each other. It was just another impromptu get-together for fun and camaraderie on the landing.

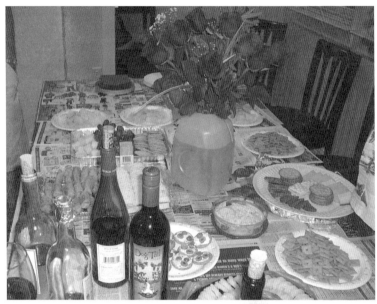

A typical table of food and wine contributed for a party. Everyone fought the battle of the bulge. Note the exquisite rose vase!

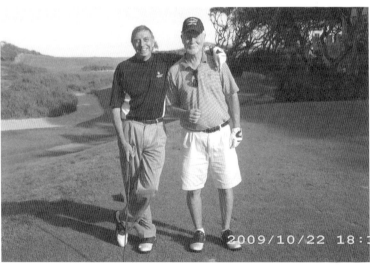

Not everything was a party. We played some golf too. The guy on the left is Bill's friend, Tom Hunter. Tom's golf partner was Tony. Both live on Amelia Island. It was a good time to see old friends and meet new ones.

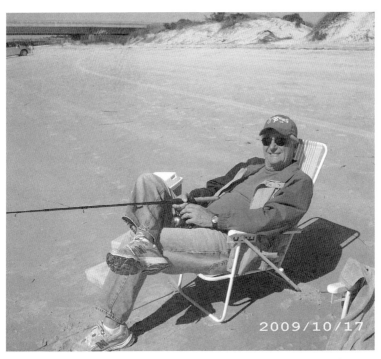

Not everything was partying and golf, there was also fishing. Catching was not so good but the sun and sand were great. We did the beach scene at least once a week.

CHAPTER 4

Clinical Studies and Investigations

One of the best ways to evaluate a particular prostate cancer therapy is to review the clinical studies and investigations related to it. Typically, these studies are reviewed and scrutinized by other researchers to ensure the methods are valid and the conclusions are backed up by the data.

There are hundreds of studies related to prostate cancer that are available on the Internet. The trick is to find good studies that address some of the questions you may have about a particular therapy. You may want to write down the questions you need to answer about the therapy you're considering. Then search for the studies that support or refute your choice.

As the authors, we were looking for research related specifically to ***proton therapy for prostate cancer***, we primarily sought out the answers to three questions: Does proton therapy work? What is proton therapy's cure rate compared to other therapies? Is proton therapy gentle or relatively nontoxic?

Following is a brief review of two studies that provided the answers to those questions. These studies and many more can be accessed via the Internet if you use a search engine and enter *Proton therapy for prostate cancer, clinical investigations or studies.*

Study Number 1:

Proton Therapy for Prostate Cancer: The Initial Loma Linda University Experience. By Jerry D. Slater, M.D., Carl J. Rossi, Jr., M.D., Les T. Yonemoto, M.D., et al.

Description of the study:

The purpose of this investigation was to analyze the results of conformal proton radiation therapy for localized prostate cancer, with emphasis on freedom from cancer relapse. This was done by using the PSA test to determine if the cancer was cured or only temporarily minimized. The results were analyzed for 1,255 patients treated at Loma Linda between October 1991 and December 1997. Results were measured primarily in terms of PSA increases and the harmful side effects that were found.

Findings:

The overall biochemical disease-free survival rate was 73 percent. It was 90 percent in patients with initial PSA of less than or equal to 4.0 when treatments were started.

It was 83 percent in patients with post-treatment PSA of less than or equal to .50.

Conclusion:

Conformal proton radiation therapy at the reported dose level yielded disease-free survival rates comparable with other forms of local therapy, with minimal morbidity.

Study Number 2:

Reduced Normal Tissue Toxicity With Proton Therapy: by James Metz, M.D., Issued from the Abramson Cancer Center of the University of Pennsylvania. Posting Date: April 28, 2002; Last Modified: June 29, 2006

Description of the study:

In this study, Dr. Metz compared the side effects of proton therapy with the side effects of conventional X-ray radiation and radical prostatectomy. The side effects of radical prostatectomy were found to have higher percentages of toxic side effects than either proton or X-ray, and couldn't be compared to either therapy directly.

Findings of the study:

Acute genitourinary (GU) toxicity was 28 to 53 percent lower with proton radiation than photon (X-ray) radiation.

Chronic impotence was 30 percent lower for proton therapy than for photon (X-ray) therapy.

Incontinence requiring a pad was less than one percent

for proton therapy as compared to 1.5 percent for photon therapy.

Conclusion:

Proton therapy is gentler to the gastrointestinal tract, and has a lower risk of impotence and incontinence than conventional photon radiation.

CHAPTER 5

The Treatment

By Bill Demboski

I usually arrived at the University of Florida Proton Therapy Institute for my daily prostate treatments about ten minutes before my scheduled time. As soon as I got there, I logged onto the computer in the lobby, which immediately let the therapists know I was there.

Shortly after my arrival, I often saw many small children arriving from the Ronald McDonald House for *their* treatments. It broke my heart to see these lovely, young children as they bravely marched into the treatment area like it was no big deal.

Because they had to remain absolutely immobile during their treatment time, the children were put under general anesthesia. Gerry Troy, our tour director, told us prostate patients that most of us had the little "c". When we saw some of the babies battling the BIG "C", we appreciated how fortunate we were.

After I'd arrived and logged in, I had about 30 minutes until my actual treatment time. At this point, a therapist came out and told me to begin drinking my water. After I'd been at the Proton Center several days, I no longer needed this reminder.

I went to a waiting station and needed to drink 16 ounces of spring water in 30 minutes, which wasn't a problem for me. The water was necessary to help inflate my bladder so it would not be in the proton path. As a result, there would be only a minimum amount of radiation to the bladder.

Later, I was greeted in the lobby area by a therapist and addressed by my last name, as a sign of courtesy. The therapist usually asked each person about their evening or weekend activities. After that, I was personally escorted into the therapy treatment area.

Once in the therapy area, I only had about 20 minutes of treatment remaining. Five or six minutes of that time involved lying on the table waiting for the proton beam. The actual proton beam time was only about 80 seconds.

Shortly after I arrived in the therapy area, 100 cc of saline solution was inserted by syringe into the rectum. The amount of the solution was so small that it was easily tolerated by most patients. This solution was needed to stabilize the prostate, to keep it within two millimeters target tolerance.

I was one of a few patients who required a balloon catheter be inserted into my rectum, then filled with 90 cc of saline, in order to stabilize my prostate to maintain the requisite two-millimeter tolerance. The rectal balloon also expands the rectum which results in less proton energy being absorbed by the rectal tissues. Fewer side effects are the result. This use of the rectal balloon caused no discomfort.

Each day the therapist who had been chosen for the rectal injections always asked me the question, "Is everything OK back there?" This became a common greeting from one patient to another—an example of our prostate cancer humor.

My treatments were scheduled in the yellow treatment station or *Gantry* as it was referred to by the medical staff. Most prostate patients were scheduled on that station (number three in the schematic below) because it was used exclusively for prostate cancer treatments. The red (number two) treatment station or gantry was used for prostate cancer treatments about 50% of the time. The overflow of prostate cancer patients and special research studies were scheduled

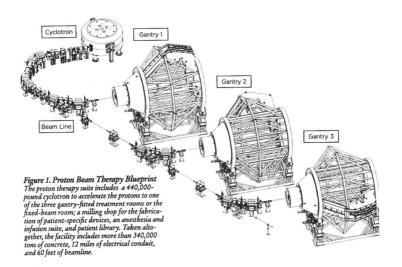

Figure 1. Proton Beam Therapy Blueprint
The proton therapy suite includes a 440,000-pound cyclotron to accelerate the protons to one of the three gantry-fitted treatment rooms or the fixed-beam room; a milling shop for the fabrication of patient-specific devices, an anesthesia and infusion suite, and patient library. Taken altogether, the facility includes more than 340,000 tons of concrete, 12 miles of electrical conduit, and 60 feet of beamline.

on the blue station (gantry number one). The blue treatment gantry was used for head, neck, and spine cancer treatments and needed significant modification to handle prostate patients. Consequently, prostate patients were treated on this gantry very early or very late in the day.

The cyclotron (proton generator) pictured above is the most expensive component of proton therapy and is shared by switching the proton beam from treatment station to treatment station.

The treatments were a breeze and I experienced no significant side effects. The biggest sin I could commit

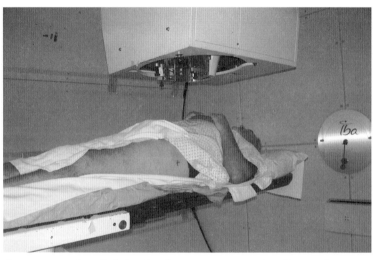

A proton patient is lying in the treatment station (gantry), preparing to receive his treatment for the day.

during a treatment was *moving*. The therapists had a two millimeter tolerance for positioning the beam, and they were very committed to those specifications. Once they had set the target to the beam, it was imperative, "**Do**

not move!" Their primary concern was the patients' well-being, and they wanted to deliver the best possible therapy results.

Because there was only one proton generator, the proton beam was switched from gantry to gantry. A significant amount of the time the patient spent on the table was waiting for the proton beam to become available for his treatment. As I mentioned before, the actual beam time was only about 80 seconds.

Usually after about the fifteenth treatment, a small ring of redness (referred to by the patients as *"therapy Badges"*) developed on both hips due to the proton energy. It was very light at first and gradually deepened in color, but it was never painful.

After 15 treatments, I did not have the *"therapy badges"* that my friend Mitch McGuire did. Gail Sarto, my nurse, said that I shouldn't worry; they would show up eventually, everyone reacted differently as far as timing was concerned. She was right. After three additional treatments the dark circles appeared.

Wednesdays were my day to see the doctor. Dr. Bill Mendenhall was my doctor during the time that I was receiving treatments and for my follow-up visits. Dr. Bill checked his ego at the door of the examination room. I felt very comfortable discussing all aspects of my therapy with him. In my case things went so well, I had very few questions. It was the easiest cancer treatment I could ever have imagined.

If I experienced any problems before my scheduled examination, I was encouraged to contact my case nurse,

Gail, anytime of the day or night. Gail was a genuine angel, easy to talk to, caring, and knowledgeable. She was someone I could discuss the most intimate topics.

Because a small portion of the urethra is in the direct path of the proton beam, everyone experiences a small amount of burning during urination. Gail suggested cranberry juice or the pill concentrate which lowers the PH of the urine, and greatly reduces the discomfort. We tried the pills and then obtained the chewable cranberry extract, which is like candy. The chewable caramel can be obtained from any vitamin or health food store and contain the equivalent of six glasses of juice. They were a staple in our treatment regimen.

On the day prior to my last treatment, I had to go to the lab in the hospital next door and have blood drawn for a PSA and free PSA test. The test results were available to the doctor and his nurse for my exit Interview the next day. My PSA was 8.3 when I came to UFPTI, and was 5.1 when I left for home. A good indicator the cancer was dying.

My exit interview was conducted by Gary Barlow. The people at the Proton Institute wanted to know how I had been treated personally and medically, and what improvements I might be able to suggest for better, faster treatments. All my comments and those of other patients were reviewed by executive staff as part of their continuous improvement process.

To see the six month test results and a list of the side effects, experienced by the authors and contributors to this book, go to the section **Patient Status Six Months**

after Treatment at the back of this book.

If you have any questions and would like to talk to me or the other writers about the proton therapy experiences, please feel free to contact us via e-mail or regular mail any time. All of those addresses are in the **Contact Information** section in the back of this book.

CHAPTER 6

Other Patients' Stories

The authors of the book thought it might be helpful to add a few personal stories written by others who received proton treatment at The University of Florida Proton Therapy Institute approximately the same time as the authors.

Gary W. Smith was raised in a very small farming community called Bennett, Iowa. Gary was diagnosed with prostate cancer in July of 2009, just after his 57th birthday. Because of his experience with self-serving urologists after his diagnosis, and hearing the horror stories of his fellow prostate patients, Gary has made it his goal to make all men aware that proton radiation is the best treatment available for low and medium Gleason score prostate cancers.

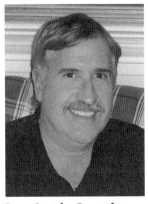

Gary Smith, Contributor

My Story by Gary Smith

I was diagnosed with Prostate Cancer (Gleason 3+3 Stage T1c) on July 20, 2009. To say that it was a shock would be the understatement of my life.

I had what is termed a *running* PSA level. Beginning in 2002, my PSA level began to rise. It had been 1.3, but jumped to 1.8 that year. In each successive year, it rose about .6 or so. Being a retired quality engineer, I know trends and this was not a good one. Finally, in June 2009, my PSA had reached 5.38. My primary doctor and I could no longer ignore it and hope for the best.

I was referred to a local urologist. He told me I should have a needle biopsy the following week. I asked if there was some other way to determine if there was cancer. He said no (which I later learned was incorrect).

The biopsy was done on July 13 in the doctor's office with no anesthesia at all, just a pain pill an hour before the procedure. The procedure was very unpleasant. The technician who was doing it kept saying, "You won't feel this one at all." I felt *every single biopsy*, 14 in all. I was told that I would have the results in three days. It turned out to be *ten* days of nervous waiting.

When I was finally called on July 20, the doctor just told me straight out that I had cancer of the prostate, and that one of the samples was 22 percent cancer. He told me that "this was the best cancer to have" because it was curable and he could place small radioactive seeds in my prostate the next week.

I asked about other treatments and he told me that

I didn't seem like a watchful, waiting sort of guy (just that *once*, he was right). Surgery would likely leave me impotent or incontinent or both and he thought that I probably didn't want to have "the hassle of 80 radiation treatments, one every day." His comment about the number of radiation treatments also turned out to be inaccurate, as the number is not nearly as high.

Besides, he said, "You are the poster boy for seed therapy. I've done over 400 of these procedures." When I asked about his data regarding side effects of the seeds, he didn't really answer. When pressed, he said that he didn't have any data. Being a data sort of guy by trade, this made me nervous, so I asked if I could get back to him the following week. I left and never went back.

With the help of my fiancé, I began to do research on the Internet. Together, we found out more than either of us really wanted to know about prostate cancer and its treatments. I made a small decision matrix with pros and cons and a real picture began to emerge. No, they don't publish statistics on side effects of the treatments for prostate cancer. However, I began to read case studies and technical papers and gleaned some data that I could use to make my decision.

Surgery was definitely not for me, as I didn't like the higher risks of impotence and incontinence (20 to 30 percent likelihood of each). I heard firsthand how this "gold standard" of treatment ruined the quality of life for many guys my age (57). I also heard that cancer could come back with this course of action. This also went along with my personal opinion (unsupported by data) that any surgical disturbance of cancer can introduce it to the lymph system, causing the spread of cancer to other organs.

I later learned that robotic surgery had even worse long-term side effects than the older, open belly surgery. The patient just didn't lose as much blood with robotic surgery.

The radioactive seed therapy had less chance of incontinence and impotence (15-20 percent) but added the risk of the seeds migrating to other areas. Ow! Accidentally irradiating my urethra or lower lungs was not a good thing to think of either. There is also a chance of passing the radioactive seeds to a sexual partner. They are currently experimenting with connecting groups of seeds to reduce migration, but they have had no luck so far.

Hormones only delayed the inevitable and had very high incidence of impotence as a side effect, so no thanks. In researching this one, it seemed as though the doctors were just charging high fees for the shots, but not telling anyone they had little effect long-term.

Photon radiation (X-rays) has been used to treat cancer for some time, but there is a lot of damage to skin and organs over time because the X-rays pass through the body with little control of depth or profile. I couldn't get enough data on the side effects of photon to come up with any *percentage* conclusions.

It seemed that conformal proton radiation beam therapy offered the lowest side effects percentages (less than one percent incontinence and 7 to 15 percent impotence, half curable over time) with a 95 percent overall cancer cure rate. The radioactive beam is targeted only to the patient's prostate and delivers the energy in a very controlled way, minimizing damage to surrounding organs, skin, and other tissue.

We also found a web site called *You Are Not Alone* (YANA) that had a nice selection of personal narratives of men who had undergone treatments for prostate cancer. I was able to glean a lot of data from those case studies.

We also found *Proton BOB*, a web site with case histories about proton treatment. At this point, I was almost convinced.

I got a second opinion from the head urologist at the University of Iowa Medical Center. He was a surgeon and said he could operate on me with minimal side effects because I was a *poster boy* for surgery. Yeah, they might be minimal to *him*, but not to *me*. By the way, doctors, keep your posters. I'm not interested.

I decided on proton therapy and contacted the Florida Proton Institute, intake services, in Jacksonville, Florida. I had a consultation and three day work-up on September 12-17. They offered me a spot in a clinical trial (hypo fractionated) treatment regimen. This a treatment consisting of 29 treatments versus the current standard 39 treatments which delivers a higher dose of proton radiation over a shorter time. The data collected so far in this trial looked good, so I accepted. Besides, 29 treatments at a higher dose, versus the current traditional regimen of 39 treatments looked attractive because it meant less time away from home and less expense for me.

I began treatment at UFPTI on October 1, 2009. While waiting for the daily treatments, I met a lot of guys who had more advanced cancer than I did. I also got to hear some real horror stories about urologists and their suggested "treatments." I heard about every conceivable combination of treatments except swinging a dead chicken over the prostate. Funny thing about us guys, when we have something like this in common, we talk and bond readily.

Each of the proton therapy treatments was sort of a nonevent. You came in, put on a hospital gown, were prepped and positioned, X-rayed to align the beam, and received protons. You couldn't feel a thing. The whole thing took about 15 minutes and you were done for the day.

Some of the guys called their days in Jacksonville *Radiation Vacation*, because we had so much free time there. I got in two days of beach time each week, went on tours of the Jacksonville area, walked and worked out every day, and found time to write. I kept up with my e-mails to the folks at home to help them to understand and not to worry. I also began to assemble a PowerPoint presentation for people back home to spread the word on this treatment option. I'm sure urologists in my hometown will hate that.

The side effects during the treatment program were minimal. I found out I had to urinate more often, partly because I was drinking a lot of water daily, and partly because the radiation irritated my prostate slightly. During my daily four mile walks, I mentally mapped all of the public rest rooms on the route. I also took a daily 220 milligram Aleve to help keep the inflammation of the prostate to a minimum.

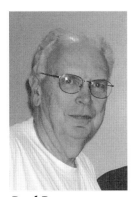

Paul Preuss,
Contributor

Paul Preuss was born in Brooklyn, New York, in 1942. Paul was diagnosed with prostate cancer in August of 2009 and received his proton treatment during October, November, and December of 2009 at UFPTI. He is eager to share his experiences of treatment and follow-up with those who are facing similar decision-making issues.

My Story by Paul Preuss

In November of 1994 my PSA was 1.0. Somewhere between then and May of 2009, it had climbed to 5.0. I have no idea regarding the steepness of its climb. Following my annual digital rectal examination (DRE), my general practitioner suggested a second prostate specific regimen (PSA) be taken. The second PSA remained at 5.0 and I was soon on my way to a urologist. He conducted a DRE, felt a nodule on the left side of my prostate, and suggested that a biopsy be taken.

The biopsy was taken on July 27 by the urologist and an assistant. Twelve cores of samples were extracted in a nearly painless fashion, although I felt some mild rectal soreness for a week or so after the procedure. Some comments made by the doctor during the biopsy and in the brief exchange at the conclusion made me sense the results would confirm cancer.

Once at home, I began a small Internet investigation

into the issues involved with prostate cancer. Therefore, I was not at all taken aback when the urologist called on August 5 at five thirty p.m. to inform me that two of the 12 cores showed positive for cancer with a Gleason score of 6.

At that point, I knew for sure that I was going to be traveling a brand new and unplanned road in my next years of retirement. A full consultation with the urologist regarding the next steps was scheduled for August 17. Here I was, at the age of 67, with a PSA of 5, a Gleason score of 6, and a brand new identity as one of the thousands with prostate cancer.

Between August 5 and August 17, my investigation into prostate cancer and the many treatment options swung into full gear, becoming an almost full-time occupation. One of the first things I decided to do was to keep a daily log of all my activities, contacts, and actions, and to also keep in this log my thoughts and reactions as they developed over time. I would strongly recommend this to all who must travel this or similar roads. You might include such details as books read, web sites visited, and key telephone numbers and e-mail addresses. You also might want to take notes regarding your findings from each source.

By the end of August 6, I had contacted all immediate family members, including my two sons and my two brothers. My eldest brother had just completed radiation therapy for cancer of the tongue. My other brother's wife was a four year survivor of stage four ovarian cancer. She is a retired teaching nurse at a major medical center in a southern state. She soon called me to see how her "cancer buddy" was doing. Frankly, I was still adjusting to the situation—and in no way did I see myself as stricken as either my eldest brother or my sister-in-law.

In one of my log postings I noted that having prostate cancer was, perhaps, similar to serving in World War II as a seaman truck driver at the docks in the Brooklyn Navy Yard. In contrast, having ovarian or tongue cancer was much more like being a Marine on Iwo Jima. Anyway, I was slowly getting used to connecting the word *cancer* with me.

By August 7, two days after receiving the formal diagnosis, I had more or less tentatively firmed up my decision to have surgery via the Da Vinci robotic surgery method. It was available at a large, nearby medical center, and it would be performed by a very highly regarded surgeon. I had actually undergone previous surgery there. This was the same surgeon that had operated on the father of our daughter-in-law, removing a cancerous bladder and creating a new one out of a section of intestine. She is still alive and healthy four years later.

My sister-in-law called to say that surgery was the "gold standard." That kind of cemented the plan in my head, but I reserved the option to change. I was still only about 90 percent sure of my surgery decision.

My research continued and I made an appointment with the surgeon for September 2, knowing that it would be difficult to gain access to him if I delayed any longer. My plan was to get my prostate issue resolved that fall, or at least before the end of the year.

Several hours before the afternoon appointment with my urologist on August 17, my wife, Becky, returned from our public library with the book *You Can Beat Prostate Cancer & You Don't Need Surgery to Do It* by Robert J. Marckini. I quickly read the book cover to cover before my appointment began.

It totally changed my point of view. The book tells the story of the author's search for "the solution" and his decision to use Proton Therapy at Loma Linda University Medical Center in California. For the first time, I became truly aware of the difference between *proton* and *photon* radiation therapy and the benefits of proton therapy over surgery.

My consultation with the urologist took place with Becky present—she took very good notes that proved valuable as a record of events which we could refer to following each such meeting. Becky helped remind me if and when I forgot to report answers to questions with sufficient detail or clarity. We were in this together,

The urologist described my cancer's stage as "soft T2". He reviewed a complete menu of options available to me, given the stage that I was at. These included watchful waiting, surgery, radiation, cryogenic treatment, and seeds.

When I mentioned my appointment with the surgeon, he mentioned that there was another surgeon in a closer community who also used robotic equipment and he offered to put me in contact with him. I declined since I had already selected the surgeon at the medical center.

When I mentioned proton beam therapy, he strongly

recommended that I speak to the local radiologist. He arranged an appointment for me before leaving his office. The urologist also put me in contact with a male RN hired by the local chapter of the American Cancer Society who was an "in house" contact for all cancer patients in the area.

My schedule for dealing with the cancer that fall was considered *reasonable* by the urologist. He said I could even wait until after the winter. I left his office, with my mind swimming with all the alternatives, but I kept coming back to proton beam therapy.

On August 18, I had a good conversation via phone with the American Cancer Society RN. He assured me that having my head swim among all the options was a natural thing, and I just had to work my way through to a decision. It was all a normal part of the process.

I spoke with a neighbor and friend who had photon radiation done locally. He was very pleased with the results—no side effects. Another neighbor, a retired MD, said that the first neighbor had one of the best results that he was aware of. I spent most of that afternoon researching more on the Internet.

By August 24, I was getting anxious and I e-mailed "Proton Bob", who runs a web site and was a prostate cancer survivor who had used the proton treatments for his cure. I asked if I should wait to contact the proton centers or go ahead immediately. The response was, "Since there's a wait time, go ahead."

I contacted three centers, one of which was the University of Florida Proton Therapy Institute. A second one was very slow to reply and they never really did complete their response to me. With the third I went as far as having a patient ID card and having an appointment, only to cancel when it became evident that there was a mismatch between what I expected and what they offered.

I found out that the head of the third facility had stated at medical symposiums that there was no difference between proton and photon therapy for prostate cancer, and indeed, proton therapy for prostate cancer was unnecessary. That did it for me. No need to go there. I canceled my appointment.

The University of Florida Proton Institute and my contact, Lisa Richardson, worked smoothly and quickly. Before I knew it, I was approved. My insurance was taken care of, and soon I was scheduled for a combination visit to handle all my intake procedures. All of this was done with fine style and care.

But, I'm getting ahead of myself. As part of my research I joined the following web groups:

www.protonbob.com "The Brotherhood of the Balloon (BOB) is a group of prostate cancer patients who have chosen conformal proton beam radiation therapy (proton treatment). The organization was formed in December 2000 by patients of the Loma Linda University Medical Center Proton Treatment Center. Today they have nearly 4,000 members representing all 50 states and 25 different countries. Support is provided by Loma Linda University Medical Center." (The specific wording was taken directly from their web site.)

www.yananow.net "Our Aim: To provide comfort to any man diagnosed with prostate cancer, to offer thoughtful support to him and his family and to help them to decide how best to deal with the diagnosis by providing them with, and guiding them to, suitable information, being mindful at all times that it is the individual's ultimate choice, that the path he decides to follow is his own and that of his family, based on his particular circumstances." (The wording was taken directly from their excellent web site).

I also perused the following web sites suggested to me by the American Cancer Society RN:

Abramson Cancer Center
www.oncolink.com

Center for Prostate Cancer Coalition
www.cpdr.com

Prostate Cancer Foundation
www.prostatecancerfoundation.org

Prostate Cancer Education Council
www.pcaw.com

The Prostate Net
www.prostate-online.org

Prostate Pointers
www.prostatepointers.org/prostate

Prostate Cancer Resource Center
www.healingwell.com/prostatecancer

Us Too
www.ustoo.com

I was also able to contact 16 former patients treated by University of Florida Proton Therapy Institute. They were eager to provide me with feedback from their experiences both at UFPTI and afterward. The book *Dr. Patrick Walsh's Guide to Surviving Prostate Cancer: Give Yourself a Second Opinion* was also a good late resource in my search for understanding. It provided many excellent details that other texts simply did not provide. Other books that were given to me were often out of date and provided incomplete information regarding proton beam therapy.

My consultation with the surgeon on September 2 went very well. He went over all the options open to me and explained the robotic procedure in depth. Since I had previous laparoscopic surgery, he indicated that my surgery would perhaps take an hour longer, a total of four hours. I told him about my interest in proton beam therapy and he shared the comments made by the head of the center that I mentioned previously—that, in effect, *proton beam therapy was not necessary.*

On September 10, I met with the local radiologist and had a useful consultation. Again, all my questions were answered in a forthright manner. When I raised the topic of proton beam radiation, those same negative comments made by the head of that one proton beam center were mentioned yet again.

Right after this consultation, I met with the RN from the American Cancer Society. He provided me with a packet of information and offered his assistance.

On the evening of September 11, I firmed up my decision to use proton beam radiation to eradicate the cancer in my prostate and to go to UFPTI to do it. The reflections from my log below indicate my feelings and thoughts at that time. I did want the cancer removed. I had investigated enough to realize that watchful waiting was not beneficial in the long run (Scandinavian studies) and so it had been discarded early on.

Refection from my log on September 15:

At this point, I feel I have accomplished all I can do in studying the various options I have to remove cancer with the minimum of after effects. All the options have after effects.

The top three options in my process are robotic radical prostatectomy (RRP), radiation at my local hospital using IMRT, and the Proton Therapy Institute in Jacksonville. I have ruled out the proton program at one facility (too long a wait) and at a second facility (too impersonal and they did not believe in the process).

Surgery was the first option to go, although I did like the surgeon and did trust his skills. It was just too hard a process with the potential of too many harsh lifelong outcomes.

Between IMRT/IGRT and proton therapy, I feel that the best chance of reduced after effects is with the protons, plus I will be in the midst of a caring environment which will include fellow patients and spouses. We will not be alone.

So, the decision has been made after much reading, talking, and research. I am satisfied with the outcome and think I have learned all I need to know to make the final determination, knowing that all is not perfect in an imperfect world. No second thoughts!

As I write this, I have completed 16 of 39 treatments at UFPTI. All has gone as expected and UFPTI has lived up to its reputation and all that I have been told about it.

Becky and I have made the most of our living in Jacksonville so far. Just about the first week we arrived, we took advantage of the reduced rates offered UFPTI patients and we joined the Jacksonville YMCA where we go three times each week. Becky likes the water aerobics and I go for lap swimming. We also obtained our Jacksonville library cards and got into the routine of checking out books and finding a branch very close to the Brooks YMCA where we swim.

We've been taking full advantage of the UFPTI schedule of Tuesday lunches and Wednesday lunch-brunch programs, although we miss out on the Thursday dinners because my treatments are typically scheduled at that time. Missing the Thursday dinners is made up for by the wine and cheese socials scheduled by the residents at the Third and Main apartments where we are staying. All of the residents are patients at the Proton Institute. We meet many great people at these events and enjoy fine discussions too.

A visit to the Jacksonville Zoo was an excellent experience as were visits to the museums of the city. We made a list and visited just about all of them. The River

Walk along both shores of the St. John's River is a great place for taking a stroll or for taking photos. Of course we enjoy our time at the beaches, our trips to the various state parks and wildlife management areas, and our excursions to places such as nearby Amelia Island and St. Augustine.

We keep a close eye on events such as the monthly Art Walk in Jacksonville, and the weekly art market on Riverside. We make the effort to check these out with the result that we find new and interesting things in each corner of this wonderful city.

Of course we have to eat, and we sample as many restaurants that fit our tastes and styles as we can, but there are so many to pick among that nine weeks is not sufficient to exhaust the list.

I find getting around Jacksonville to be rather simple once I got the road system down and having a detail map did help. The city has a good system of interconnecting highways and bridges and we are able to travel good distances in relatively short amounts of time with ease once we learned the way.

We also find shopping to be a good way to spend some of our time, both out of necessity and just for fun. The large St. John's City Center is one of our more frequent destinations for both shops and restaurants. There's no need to fear *not* having enough to do in Jacksonville, and I haven't even mentioned golf!

I cannot share what lies ahead. That is for others to tell. But I have no doubt that this is the right place for me and that my decision making process was sound as was the outcome of the process.

I learned that, for the most part, the medical profession does not know about proton beam therapy. I learned that doctors at home really wanted to keep me at home, if at all possible. I wonder what my reception will be when I return. No doubt, I will be accepted but perhaps not as welcome as I attempt to lead others down the proton pathway.

I really think that, in the future, surgery will be a thing of the past for this disease. I believe proton radiation, or its derivatives, will replace X-ray Radiation. Costs will control for awhile, until proton equipment gets smaller and less expensive. We are just seeing the first generations and more are coming along with even greater capacities. What is the newest and best today will soon be old in a few tomorrows. Such is the nature of this technology. I feel fortunate to have been able to come to UFPTI at this period of my life.

*   *   *

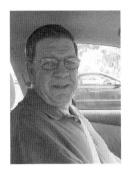

Bill Norrell,
Contributor

William (Bill) Norrell was born in Chattanooga, Tennessee, in 1942. Bill was diagnosed with prostate cancer in 2009. His contribution to this book was to help men understand that the proton treatment for prostate cancer is a great option for maintaining your quality of life and usually is not mentioned by your urologist. It was the best option for Bill.

My Story by Bill Norrell

My nightmare began on January 1, 2009. I called my wife to check on some blood clots floating in the toilet. We decided to go to the emergency room (ER) in the hospital near our home.

After CT scans and blood and urine tests which came out negative, the physician in the emergency room told me that there was a possibility I was passing a kidney stone. He advised me to go to a urologist.

We left the ER and went back home. From then on my health started to change for the worse.

I soon started to feel weak in my legs. I remembered I was taking pills for my high blood pressure, but I didn't think these could be causing the problem.

A few days later another blood clot was found in my urine. This time I panicked. All my tests had come back negative after the first occurrence. Even my PSA's and DRE's were normal, so whatever was causing these problems was a grave concern.

We went back for the second time to the ER and they repeated the same tests. At this point I was aggravated and very upset. Another physician from the ER told me that all the test results were negative, and they could not find the source of the blood.

We then called a urologist for an appointment. I had a PSA test, a digital rectal examination (DRE), and a Cystoscopy was performed to rule out prostate problems, kidney stones, and bladder cancer. All the results were normal including a PSA of 1.9 mg/dl. The urologist told me if I experienced the same symptoms again, I should go to my primary physician and get examined.

I was still getting very weak. Two weeks later I told my wife I was feeling dizzy and needed to go to the ER. We called an ambulance because I did not want to wait for hours in the emergency room lobby. I wanted to be seen by a physician right away. I had the same tests performed and all the results were negative. We were desperate with no answers to our questions.

Three months passed, with me going back and forth to hospitals and doctors' offices, and we still didn't have a clue what was wrong. I spoke with my cousin about my conditions and he said that he was having some of the same symptoms and was passing blood in his urine. All his test results also came out negative. No one in the VA hospital could find out what was wrong with him, so he went to the Mayo Clinic. They found out what was wrong with him and he was treated for his condition. He told me that I also needed to go to the Mayo Clinic.

In the meantime, I had another bout of passing blood and weakness. Before we got to the ER, I started to feel better. I looked at my wife and I told her that this was a good time to go to the Mayo Clinic.

We arrived at the Mayo Clinic ER that Saturday and they immediately did a urine culture. It came back with a serious urinary tract infection (UTI) and they placed me on an IV antibiotic immediately. They made an appointment with a urologist for the following Monday.

The urologist checked my prostate and everything seemed to be normal. The PSA was 2.1 mg/dl and the DRE was smooth. They found that the medicines I'd been previously prescribed, Flomax and Levaquin, were causing a bad interaction with the blood pressure medicine I was taking. They treated me with another antibiotic and this one seemed to work fine.

I felt ill a few days later and went back to our area hospital on the advice of my primary physician. There they ordered an IVP (a test to check kidney function for obstructions) and blood tests again. Nothing was abnormal.

I received a call from the Mayo Clinic and they recommended I have the TURP (transurethral resection of the prostate) done because they found my prostate was swollen. This was constricting the urethra and that was why I was developing the symptoms of urinary tract infections, weakness, dizziness, and bleeding. The TURP was performed and I was discharged from the Mayo Clinic Hospital two days after surgery.

We went back home and five days later my urologist

from Mayo called me with the bad news that a few tissues that were removed from the prostate had come out positive for cancer. This "C" word really struck my wife and me very hard. We never thought that after going through so many physicians and hospital visits, the result was going to be cancer.

The next step was prostate biopsies to check if the cancer was around the prostate or encapsulated. Ten biopsies were taken and all were negative. The result of the pathology report from the TURP was, I had cancer. It was rated cancer stage T1A. Mine was in the early stage and Gleason 6, not highly aggressive. I needed to do something.

They suggested "watchful waiting," something that didn't convince me at all. I also did not want surgeries, seeds, or any other traditional methods.

Through my wife's dentist, we came to learn about the University of Florida Proton Therapy Institute in Jacksonville, Florida. We looked into this, and found out that, without a doubt, this therapy was going to be the best option for me.

We contacted UFPTI and filled out the required paperwork. They sent us a script for blood work for a PSA, a Free PSA, and an alkaline phosphate test. The people at the Proton Institute contacted me to come in and do the three day work-up and gave me a starting date for treatments.

Indeed, now that I am almost finishing my treatment, I can say that this was the best decision I have ever made in regard to my prostate cancer. I've always said to everyone that I've met—*it's **your** choice, not your physician's or anyone else's to make. Always check out your options. If you do, I am quite sure you will choose, as I did, proton therapy. You can have your treatments and maintain your quality of life with few or no side effects at all.*

Hooray for proton therapy is all I can say!

*   *   *

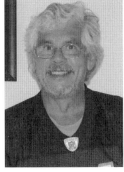

Dan Cibock was born on January 31, 1955, in Chicago, Illinois. Dan was diagnosed with prostate cancer in 2009. His goal is to help others determine the right option for treatment. His best option was proton therapy.

**Dan Cibock,
Contributor**

My Story by Dan Cibock

Well, where do I begin telling about my prostate cancer and proton therapy? I guess, at the beginning.

I had gone in for a routine checkup by my family doctor in early April of 2009. The following week, I was in Charleston, South Carolina. When I returned, I had a message on the machine, as well as a card in the mail with a message that I was to call my doctor as soon as possible for a follow-up visit. I thought to myself, "*Damn! He's going to complain about my cholesterol level—**again**!*"

I had already prepared myself for this discussion. I had really been watching my diet and had been exercising on a daily basis since last August. In fact, I was in my best physical shape in years. I had dropped 75 pounds and was feeling great. My daily run/walk was five miles long. Aside from losing weight, I felt great. I really had no idea what he was going to tell me.

When the doctor entered the room, he didn't mince words. He told me that my PSA score was 5.7, compared to 3.2 two years ago. Being naive, I asked him what that all meant. He told me that I either had a case of Prostatitis or prostate cancer.

I felt the life draining from me, just because of that word *cancer*. I was glad I was sitting down for that bit of news.

The doctor said that he would write me a prescription for an antibiotic, but he would also refer me to a local urologist after this course of medication. I was devastated!

After the week on meds, I met for the first time with the urologist. Bedside manner was not this doctor's strong suit. He concurred with my family doctor that I could just have a case of Prostatitis, but more than likely it was prostate cancer. He gave me a script for a stronger antibiotic and we scheduled another visit at the conclusion of that run. He also ordered another PSA test run, and this time, he also wanted a free PSA. He went on to explain that in all likelihood, I had prostate cancer. It almost seemed that he relished the possibility.

He then proceeded to explain my four options: 1) If I only expected to live another five to seven years, I could do nothing 2) Have surgery to remove the prostate gland 3) Undergo eight weeks of X-ray radiation 4) Undergo four weeks of X-ray radiation plus the implant of radioactive seeds.

The good doctor also told me about some of the side effects that *can* occur in some patients. Yee gads! Those side effects, in themselves, were scary!

My follow-up visit to the urologist all but confirmed his prostate cancer diagnosis, but there were two other procedures that he wanted me to undergo. The first was a biopsy of the gland, and the second was a bone scan, to see if my cancer had spread from the gland.

The biopsy was positive for cancer, but the good news was that it had not spread outside of the prostate. My Gleason score was 3+3=6.

Once the results from these last two tests were received, I again met with the urologist. As he reminded me, we were getting close to decision time, as to which of the three procedures we would follow. I had already ruled out surgery, having read and heard too many horror stories. I was leaning toward the radiation/seed implant route, but to help me make up my mind, the doctor referred me to a radiologist-oncologist. He also gave me a book to read which was thicker than *War and Peace*. I took that Friday off, went to the beach, and read the book from cover to cover.

In the meantime, I was talking to a friend of mine with whom I had worked for 30 years and told him what I was facing. He told me about one of his close friends, one with whom I had golfed several times over the years. That friend also had prostate cancer, and he had it treated with a newer, noninvasive procedure in Jacksonville, Florida. I needed to know more.

I called this gentleman that evening. He had completed his treatment earlier, in January of 2009. He told me all about his condition and how he researched everything to make his decision on his course of treatment. He had asked if my urologist had mentioned proton therapy as an option. When I told him *no*, he wasn't surprised. Neither had his.

He suggested that I go on-line and read about the University of Florida Proton Therapy Institute, in Jacksonville. That evening, I went on the web site and read everything that I could. I also requested the information packet, which arrived early the following week.

My meeting with the radiologist-oncologist was less than stellar. Here again, the bedside manner chapter must have been skipped over in his medical school. He went on to tell me how qualified he was to administer the X-ray radiation treatment or the radiation/seed implant process and I was the perfect candidate for either. He did the best he could to steer me away from surgery, but also explained to me about the possible side effects of all three procedures.

When I asked if he had ever heard of proton radiation treatments, his whole mannerism changed. He said, "Well, it's viewed as new, maybe cutting edge, and kind of *sexy!*" Both of his hands were raised in the air. "And, all that procedure will do is add a bunch of dollars to your treatment costs!" After that 15 second exchange, he changed the subject completely.

With the information packet arriving from Jacksonville, Florida, I had another book to read—*You Can Beat Prostate Cancer* by Bob Marckini. I took that Friday off and went to the beach to read again.

My next appointment was that following Tuesday with the urologist. When he came in, he bluntly asked me what course of treatment I had chosen. I told him that I had read the book that he had given me and told him, quite frankly, that it scared the living Hell out of me.

He again asked for my decision. I told him that I had made a decision. I reminded him of our initial conversation, in which he told me that he would refer me to any facility that I wanted (for surgery). I told him that I wanted him to forward my file to the Proton Therapy Institute in Jacksonville. He looked at me (I'll never forget his glare) and said that he had heard very little about it, didn't know their address, and then he curtly suggested that I needed to research this further.

I told him that I had done research and that I had talked to a couple of former patients. When I had gotten the information from Florida, and after I had read Bob Marckini's book, I had sent Bob an e-mail. He replied and sent me a five page spreadsheet with names of proton therapy graduates, three of whom I had contacted.

The doctor looked at me again and said, "Well, I don't even know their address!" I stared back at him, handing him the two page information request form. I told him that that was why I had made a copy.

I caught him completely off guard. I also told him that I was a young man, 54, and didn't want to endure all the complications I'd heard about or read about with other treatments. I said, "I don't want to be in my backswing and suddenly piss my pants. I also don't want to wear a diaper for several months or risk the possibility of being impotent, short-term or long-term.

He grabbed the form from me and started rifling through my file. He said that they would forward my records and biopsy slides to UFPTI. Then, he abruptly left the office. I thanked him as he was leaving. What was the icing on the cake? It took his office over two weeks to forward my files to Jacksonville! You know, it was ironic that the reactions of the urologist and the radio-oncologist were almost exactly what Bob Marckini had encountered and described in his book.

So, the obvious next step was to check with my insurance company. Surprisingly enough, my treatment would be covered. In early September, I went to Jacksonville for my week of work-ups, which also included finding a place to stay for my eight week *radiation vacation*. Once I found my new home, everything just fell into place.

My first treatment was Wednesday, September 23. Even though the processes and procedures were fully explained to me during that work-up week, I still didn't know, for sure, exactly what to expect. All I can say is that the entire staff at Jacksonville has been just great to work with, and to be associated with. I knew early on that the choice was the right one for me.

Monday, November 9, was my thirty-second treatment out of 39. At no time have I ever second-guessed my decision, which I am very good at doing sometimes.

In my opinion, this is the *only* course of treatment for prostate cancer. During my free time between treatments, which was quite extensive, I enjoyed the sightseeing, happy hours, and parties. I've thought to myself many times, "*Prostate cancer treatment was the source of more fun than I ever expected!*"

CHAPTER 7

A Funny Thing Happened to Us on the Way to Prostrate Cancer Treatment

Every Wednesday there is a luncheon sponsored by the Proton Institute. It's for all patients, new patients, alumni, and patients who have completed the treatments (graduates), plus friends of patients or anyone interested in hearing what is being said about the Proton Institute or the treatments. It is a great source of information and many friendships are forged from the casual comments and chance meetings. I would recommend everyone who chooses the proton option attend these lunches every chance they get. It is one of the things that the UFPTI does that makes everyone feel connected and not isolated.

Everyone who wants to speak and offer comments or relate an experience is given the microphone and many funny stories are told. This chapter is dedicated to all the phenomenal proton patients and their great senses of humor. They made us all laugh while sharing their funny insights about prostate cancer treatments. The therapists were also funny and had retorts for any remarks we made to try to shock them.

Gary Smith's Special Night Light

Gary Smith was a contributor to this book. He was on the accelerated treatment program in Jacksonville. This shortened program was being tested to determine through clinical trials if the length of treatment could be shortened from the normal 39 days to just 29 days.

During the 29 day program, Gary received more radiation during each treatment than those of us who were involved in the normal program. One day we were sitting around enjoying some adult beverages at one of our get-togethers and someone asked Gary if he felt any different. He responded by saying that he didn't feel any differently ... but with all the lights out, he could still read the paper by the light coming from his glowing *member*.

The McGuire Twins

At the beginning of September, Mitch and Lois's son and daughter-in-law came to Jacksonville for a visit, along with their twin granddaughters.

One day the girls accompanied Lois and Mitch to the Proton Institute for daily treatment. The facility has a very nice playroom for children, and the girls were happy there.

When Mitch came into the playroom before his treatment, the girls urged Mimi (that's what they called Lois) to leave the playroom and go with *Poppy*. One of the girls explained, "Mimi, we saw that sign that said **Unattended Children Will Be Given a Cup of Espresso and a Free Puppy**."

The two girls had deduced that if they were left alone, they would get a free puppy and a cup of coffee. A sip of coffee was one of their favorite things. Their only concern was whether they could get *two* free puppies or just *one*. They reasoned that, even if they were *twin* sisters, they weren't the *same people*. Therefore, in their minds, two puppies were possible.

Needless to say, the girls' visit did wonders for both Mitch and Lois's spirit.

Ramon, the therapist

Bill was in his last week of treatment and was in a happy mood. All had gone well and he had no side effects. As he climbed up on the treatment table on the last day, he told Ramon, "I hear they fill the balloons with champagne on the last day as a special treat for the patient."

Ramon, without missing a beat, said, "Yes, we do. We also pump the balloon up so the patient can taste the bubbly."

This wasn't a pleasant thought, but we all had a great laugh.

Frisky Tom Enright

Tom and Sandy Enright were from Kennett Square, Pennsylvania. They had several common friends with Bill, who was also from that neck of the woods. Tom was about four weeks ahead of Bill in treatments. Tom and Bill partied together and drank copious amounts of wine.

On Wednesday of each week there was a free luncheon at the Proton Institute. It was intended for all patients, friends of patients, and interested parties. During each luncheon the alumni, the graduates, and the new patients were introduced.

Tom wasn't shy about talking up the merits of proton therapy. When it was his turn, he stood up and told everyone that he experienced no side effects, although some people had told him he would experience some temporary sexual dysfunction. Then he announced to all, "Since Sandy and I came to Jacksonville, *we've been like two bunnies!*"

Sandy just about crawled under the table during the thunderous applause that followed. (Incidentally, Sandy was a librarian in her former life.)

Gerry Troy

Gerry Troy, MSW, administrator of patient services, was the person who ran the weekly luncheons. Gerry was sharp-witted and always had a few stories or one-liners that garnered a good laugh. No one could tell a story with impeccable delivery and timing like Gerry.

One Wednesday we were all standing and sitting around preparing for the discussion when Gerry held up the first digit on his right hand and asked the group, "What's this?" as he held his finger up high. Naturally, one of the men yelled out, "A digital exam!" Then Gerry held two fingers up and asked the same question. Hearing no response, Gerry said, "Second opinion."

The Lonely Patient

Most of the patients were fortunate to have their wives with them, and that certainly made their stays in Jacksonville feel more like home. Gerry told the story about a patient who was at the Proton Institute alone and often commented how he missed his wife *so* much. To alleviate his feeling of loneliness while sleeping, he decided to shave one of his legs. As the hair grew back on his shaved leg, stubble appeared. After that, each turn in bed made him feel like he was with his wife, and the loneliness passed.

Everyone had a good laugh until Gerry shared the rest of the story. One patient who had heard this fabricated story, a story which was meant for humorous respite, had taken it a bit too seriously. He announced at the luncheon several weeks after hearing the story that he had shaved his leg—and GOLLY! It worked!

Butt Pictures

Each time a patient climbed up on the treatment table, one of two things would happen depending on which was the more effective way to stabilize the prostate. Either 100 cc of saline solution was inserted into the rectum, or a small balloon inflated with 90 cc of saline solution was inserted. This was done to stabilize the prostate while the treatment was in progress.

Therefore, the patient entered the treatment area wearing an open end hospital gown. He then climbed up on the table and lay on his side. One of the therapists was designated as the "butt processor" for each patient. That honor rotated among the therapists in a way we patients never quite figured out.

Some patients were friendlier with the therapist than others, and had an ongoing friendly banter during each treatment. If the therapist was feeling particularly humorous and it was close to Halloween, he/she might write *BOO* on the cheeks of the patient's butt with a magic marker. Another time, the therapist might write a large "W" on each cheek so when the patient bent over it spelled *WOW*. Sometimes, patients had a "U" on one cheek and an "F" on the other.

When a proton patient was receiving his last treatment, he might get a GOOD LUCK, one word on each cheek. If their name was BOB—well, use your imagination. Sometimes patients received stick-on stars or flags. We loved it!

Mr. M from North Carolina

Mr. M was an older, well-spoken, impeccably dressed, well-educated black man. Mr. M always had a smile on his face and would talk to anyone in a heartbeat.

One day Bill and Mr. M were sitting in the lobby waiting for their treatment call. In casual conversation, Bill asked Mr. M what he did on the weekends. This topic of conversation was commonplace, since everybody was looking for good places to sightsee or restaurants to patronize.

Mr. M told Bill that he drove home every weekend, a 550 mile trip one way. Bill asked him why he felt he was required to travel such long distances every weekend.

Mr. M's response was, "But you don't understand. My wife is still working and she is 20 years younger than me. I told her the reason I was going so far for prostate treatment was the lack of negative side effects and I have to go home every week to prove I made the right choice."

There were about eight other people listening to our conversation, and when he delivered the punch line, the place exploded with laughter. Needless to say, after each visit, Mr. M was asked, "So, how's everything working these days?"

Mr. M was a real sport about the needling we gave him.

The Halloween Party

Vivian and Bill Norrell were the Third and Main organizers. They would come up with ideas and then do most of the work to make them happen. One day we were sitting around the breezeway and Vivian said, "We should have a Halloween Party and we can make costumes optional. I will make a flier and put it on every door so everyone knows they are invited." The stage was set.

We encouraged everyone to get some type of makeshift costume because the purpose was a good time and no judging would occur. If you reference the pictures in the book you can see some of the clever costumes that were conceived.

It shows what imagination can do when you need a Halloween costume and don't want to spend much money.

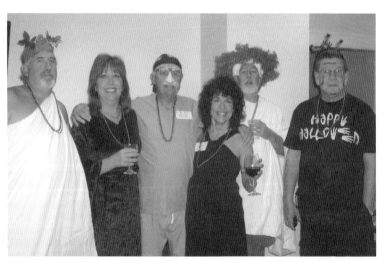

Everyone thought Bill Zeallear was the most innovative costume maker with the use of a Christmas Wreath as a replacement for a crown of laurel. Needless to say, everyone had a great time and saw firsthand that prostate cancer was a source of more fun than we ever expected.

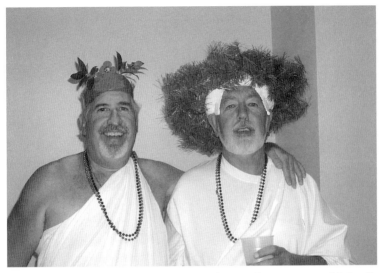

Gary Smith and Bill Zeallear were the two live wires and life of the party. "Girls, please do not take candy from either of these two men."

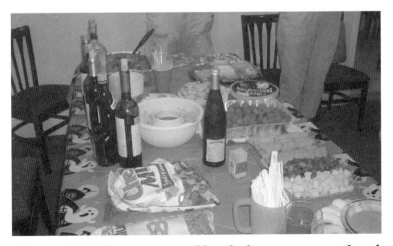

This was the Halloween party table, which every one contributed to. Believe me, no one went hungry or lacked for drinks. Bill and Vivian Norrell posted invitation signs and did all the decorations. They also set up the beautiful table with all the goodies.

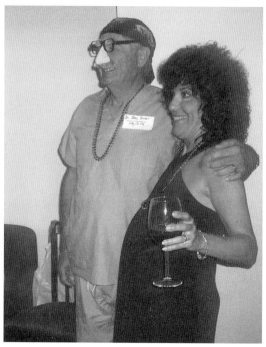

Doctor Ben Dover, OBGYN, played by Bill Demboski and his pretend pregnant patient, played by Karen Demboski.

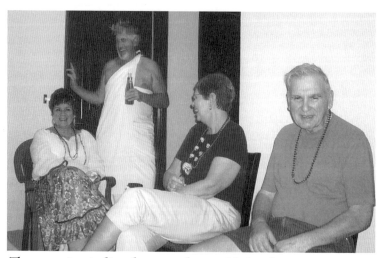

The party is winding down on the outside landing.

A Texas Tale

Karen and Bill attended the weekly lunch at the Proton Institute during Bill's six-month checkup. During the lunch, Ray Easter, who was completing the treatments that day, shared the following story.

Before the first treatment all patients are a little apprehensive. This was the case with Ray as he waited in the foyer to be escorted for his first treatment. Ray and his wife, Phyllis, were sitting waiting for his turn. Sitting next to Ray was a patient from Texas who said to Ray, "Don't worry about the treatment. It's a breeze!" This relieved Ray's anxiety and they began to chat. Since the Texan was soon to graduate, he was an expert on all aspects of the therapy. He asked Ray, "Are you getting the 29 or 39 treatments?" Ray, being new to the therapy, asked what the difference was. The Texan answered, "Both work, but the doctors have found that with each treatment your "*Willie*" grows by a 1/8 inch." With that information offered, Phyllis tapped Ray on the knee and said, ***"Go for the 39 treatments!"***

CHAPTER 8

Frequently Asked Questions

Question 1: What is the contact information for the University of Florida Proton Therapy Institute?
Answer: Call toll free (877) 686-6009 or go on-line to www.floridaproton.org.

Question 2: What is the cost of proton therapy treatments?
Answer: The cost will vary depending on the patient's age, the rank of his disease, the length of his treatment, and his insurance. In the case of each of the authors, the cost was zero because their insurance covered it entirely. Author Bill Demboski's cost, *without* insurance, would have been $160,000 for his 39 treatments. The Proton Center has a financial resource advisor, Denise Sikes, who works with prospective patients and explores the options for payment. She does all the necessary calling

and researching to determine the exact reimbursements and costs. The government currently allows one to deduct travel expenses and apartment costs while under medical treatment.

Question 3: Are there any other proton centers in the United States besides the facility in Jacksonville, Florida?

Answer: There are currently seven operating in the United States: one in Loma Linda, California; Massachusetts General Hospital; Indiana University; Jacksonville; Houston, Texas; Oklahoma City, and the University of Pennsylvania. There are a total of 22 proton centers worldwide. Four centers are currently under construction in the United States and one will be added at the University of Miami in the next few years. There are 12 additional centers under construction worldwide.

Question 4: If you had to select the best sources to learn more about proton therapy for prostate cancer, what would they be?

Answer: Following is a list of valuable sources of information:

A) The best source, by far, is surviving prostate cancer patients who have experienced proton therapy firsthand. An excellent source to connect with proton patients is the **Brotherhood of the Balloon** at www.protonbob.com. After going to the site, you can sign up for a list of 50 patients and their phone numbers, so you can talk to them personally.

B) The book entitled, *You Can Beat Prostate Cancer and You Don't Need Surgery to Do It* (ISBN 978-0-6351-4022-3) by Bob Marckini contains a wealth of information including statistics on other prostate cancer therapies.

C) Contact the University of Florida Proton Therapy Institute (UFPTI) in Jacksonville, Florida, and ask them for an information package. If you'd like, you can visit them in person and ask questions. You may also attend one of their free Wednesday luncheons and listen to current patients talk about their experiences.

D) The book by Bradley Hennenfent M.D., entitled *Surviving Prostate Cancer without Surgery* (ISBN 978-09717454-1-4).

E) The Internet. The problem with the Internet, of course, can be the amount of time it takes to sift through the massive amounts of available material.

F) Network with others. Let people know that you have been diagnosed with prostate cancer and you want to talk to others that have been through various therapies. It will surprise you how many people will tell you their stories. Listen and don't be afraid to ask pointed questions.

G) The American Cancer Society. If you contact them through the Internet, they will send you a lot of information.

H) Local seminars, usually those conducted by local urologists. Remember, some of these doctors may have some financial interest in a local treatment center and may be trying to drum up some business. Each doctor is likely to have his individual biases, which must be considered when listening to his remarks and recommendations.

These seminars provide an opportunity to network with others who are looking for answers regarding prostate cancer.

Question 5: How many men will find out that they have prostate cancer each year?

Answer: The American Cancer Society estimates that there were 221,000 new cases in 2009. About one in six men will get prostate cancer in his lifetime. Approximately 29,000 men will die from the disease this year.

Question 6: What are the most likely side effects of proton therapy and what is the probability of each?

Answer: Neither of the male authors of this book experienced any side effects following proton therapy treatment. Two sources we've summarized in Chapter 4 will also shed some light on this subject: First, a paper written by Dr. James Metz entitled *Reduced Tissue Toxicity with Proton Therapy*. Second, a clinical investigation paper from Loma Linda entitled *Proton Therapy for Prostate Cancer*.

Question 7: What would you consider the biggest downside of proton therapy?

Answer: If the Proton Center isn't close to home, a patient would have to spend approximately two months away from home. If he's still working, that would result in a loss of income. Also, housing arrangements would have to be made for that period of time.

Question 8: For what reason might a cancer patient be rejected from receiving proton therapy?
Answer: Patients who are in poor health, advanced in age, or have a series of complications from medical problems, may not be qualified. Each patient is evaluated thoroughly by the medical staff and each case, depending on the patient needs and health issues, is evaluated by the medical staff before a decision is made to treat or decline.

Question 9: Do you have any statistics dealing with cure rates?
Answer: Getting a handle on cure rates is difficult. It depends on the aggressiveness of the prostate cancer, how early it was diagnosed, the health of the patient, and his compliance to treatment. In 30 to 50 percent of the cases, the cancer extends beyond the gland itself. If you consider the cases that are not particularly aggressive and are diagnosed early, proton therapy cure rates can be as high as 97 percent, as confirmed by a study in 2008 (JAMA, Zeitman). If you take a look at all the therapies for prostate cancer, they have about the same cure rates. The big difference between the therapies is the number of negative side effects. If you study all the therapies, the one with the fewest side effects is proton therapy.

Question 10: Is proton therapy used to treat other types of cancers?
Answer: Yes, there are treatment protocols for neck, spine, head, eye, pancreatic, soft tissue, genitourinary, lung,

pediatric, and brain. Other protocols are being developed for kidney, breast, and other soft tissue carcinomas.

Question 11: What do you consider the biggest downside of prostate cancer treatments?

Answer: While the cancer can be cured, terrible side effects may affect the quality of life. Sexual dysfunction, incontinence, and colitis like symptoms are major concerns.

Question 12: Of all prostate cancers that are diagnosed, what percent of them are detected early, have not migrated from the gland, and are considered early-stage?

Answer: About 80 percent of men diagnosed have early-stage cancer.

Question 13: Is proton therapy considered experimental?

Answer: Proton therapy is not an experimental treatment. It has been used to treat cancer tumors since 1954 and has had a commercial history of treatment since 1990 when Loma Linda, California, opened and began treating patients. Since 1954, 50 thousand patients have been treated with proton beam radiation.

Question 14: Which cancer patients make the best candidates?

Answer: Proton therapy is most effective in cancers that have not spread through the bloodstream to other sites in the body.

Question 15: Will my insurance cover proton therapy?

Answer: Medicare and most major insurance carriers in the United States cover proton therapy.

Question 16: How long does proton therapy treatment take?

Answer: The actual time in the treatment station (gantry) each day is 15 to 45 minutes. The proton beam is delivered to the patient for one minute of that time. The standard therapy consists of 39 treatments, but trials are in progress to determine if the treatments can be reduced to 29 with higher doses of proton radiation for each treatment. Most patients receive one treatment per day.

Question 17: Can proton therapy be used in conjunction with other cancer treatments?

Answer: Yes, patients with cancer often undergo more than one type of therapy. Proton can be used in combination with conventional X-ray radiation, chemotherapy, and surgery.

Question 18: How many patients can the Florida Proton Center treat each day?

Answer: They are able to treat up to 150 patients a day.

Question 19: What does it cost to build a typical proton treatment center?

Answer: The demand for proton therapy is increasing, with several new centers being constructed worldwide. Local physicians aren't building proton treatments centers because the initial costs are between 150 and 200 million dollars. Also, a staff of physicists is necessary to maintain beam transmission and quality.

Question 20: Is the University Of Florida Proton Therapy Institute a for-profit facility?

Answer: No, the center is a nonprofit organization dedicated to improving patients' quality of life. The University of Florida administers gifts and donations designated for the center. This funding is used to support construction and clinical research. One-third of all profits of this book will be donated to UFPTI for clinical research.

CHAPTER 9

A Local Urologist Discredits Proton Therapy

By Bill Demboski

On Tuesday, January 26, 2010, Karen and I decided to attend a prostate cancer seminar at a local, well-known urologist's office. The seminar was well-advertised, and Karen and I expected a good turnout.

About 36 people attended, mostly couples. Many of the males in attendance had recently learned that they had prostate cancer.

During the entire seminar, I took copious notes. All of the following observations I made were corroborated by my wife.

Much of the information that the doctor shared involved things that we'd learned previously during our cancer research. Most of the information he provided was accurate, but there were some glaring exceptions.

He described five methods of treating prostate cancer:
1. Watchful waiting
2. Hormone therapy
3. Photon radiation (X-ray)
4. Surgery
5. Cryosurgery

After his presentation, and during the question and answer period, I asked the doctor why he didn't mention proton radiation as an option. His response was, "Why? Did I miss one?"

The response seemed a little arrogant since the advertisement specifically said participants would be learning ALL the latest prostate cancer treatments and new advances.

The doctor then stated, "Proton therapy doesn't work! Although I have not seen clinical data on side effects, my experience is that they're very high ... *much* higher than IMRT radiation."

He then went on to claim that he had nine patients who went to Jacksonville, Florida, to the University of Florida Proton Therapy Institute. Five of those were unhappy with the side effects.

He also told the audience that Medicare and most insurance plans would not pay for the treatment. He indicated that proton therapy was very expensive, and since it didn't really work, he would not recommend the treatment.

"But go ahead if you're rich and can afford the treatment!" he said. "It's your money!"

He then stated that there were 12 to 16 proton

treatment centers in operation or being built. Karen and I looked at each other and said, "Why would they be building all these centers if the treatment doesn't work?"

We were ready to walk out!

No one in the audience asked any additional questions about proton therapy with that kind of *expert* opinion offered by such a prominent doctor.

It became obvious to Karen and me that the losses of income by the local doctors when the patient chooses proton therapy was a driving force behind his recommendation. If he wanted to learn about the effectiveness of proton treatment, all the information and clinical studies are available to the medical world on cure rates and side effects. One hour on the Internet would educate him on the treatment modality and the number of patients successfully treated each year.

Karen and I are convinced that it's all about the doctors who treat cancer losing control of the MONEY. As of the date of this book's publication, there have been approximately 60,000 patients successfully treated with proton therapy.

If it didn't work, why are patients continuing to have it done—and why is the medical community building more treatment centers around the world?

About the Four Coauthors

Bill Demboski

William (Bill) Demboski was born in Justus, Pennsylvania, in 1936. He attended St. James Catholic High School for Boys. After serving four years in the United States Navy, Bill eventually graduated from Widener University with a degree in electronics engineering.

Bill worked in a number of small companies to obtain corporate experience. He began his career in the medical parts department of the DuPont Company. After serving numerous supervisory and management positions for 25 years, he retired in 1996, to become a self-taught artist.

In 2003 he moved to Sarasota, Florida. There he met and married Karen Marcey, a transplant from Boston, Massachusetts. Their children and grandchildren live in the Northeast, with the cold and snow. Between Bill and Karen they have four daughters and seven grandchildren, with one more on the way.

Bill likes to play golf, hunt, and fish. He dabbles in wildlife art and photography.

Karen Demboski

Karen was born into an Italian American family, and raised in Maynard, Massachusetts, a small town about 20 miles west of Boston. Educated locally, she worked as a dental office manager for many years.

She then turned her attention to retail management and design. Karen managed many women's clothing stores under several different corporate cultures and operational management styles. She also created and developed a wedding consultant business.

After that, Karen had the good sense to find her place in the sun with her late husband, John. After John's passing, she continued her retail career and created a craft business with her longtime friend, Penny, who had also migrated to Sarasota, Florida, from the Maynard area.

Karen met and fell in love with Bill Demboski and married him when she found out he could cook. They enjoy traveling, theater, sunny beaches, and their blended family of children and grandchildren.

Mitchell G. McGuire, Jr.

Mitchell is a native of Lexington, North Carolina. He holds a BA in behavioral science with certification in mathematics from Kean University.

After he graduated from college, Mitchell was a junior engineer with Walter Kiddie Co, Inc. He worked as a high school mathematics teacher, and was the first African American manager of Howard Johnson Restaurant Company, Inc.

Mitchell then began a long career in law enforcement. After many years of commendable service, he retired from the Newark Police Department in 1997 with the rank of captain/acting deputy chief. His career path in law enforcement spanned many areas, including commanding the detective bureau, intelligence, the training division, and the internal affairs bureau. During his career, he received numerous community and departmental awards, in addition to more than 200 commendations.

After retirement, Mitchell served as director of professional standards and investigations for the New Jersey Transit Police until resigning in May 2000 to become an owner and operator of a McDonald's restaurant. He has owned several McDonald's restaurants in Newark, and currently owns two in Jersey City, where he employs more than 100 of the community's young people.

Mitchell and his wife, Lois, have two children: Mitchell III, a systems engineer, and Michale, who is the director of operations of the family business. Mitchell and Lois have three grandchildren.

Today, he is the past president of the New York/New Jersey Metro Black McDonald's Operator Association. The New York Metro chapter is one of 21 chapters throughout the United States making up the NBMOA, which is a national self-help organization. It was established for the purpose of working together for the improvement and betterment of every member of the McDonald's family and the community as a whole. He also serves on various boards and community help organizations. He works tirelessly to encourage, employ, and develop the youth of his community.

Lois McGuire

Lois G. McGuire took an early retirement after 25 years in senior level human resources management. Her career included all phases of human resources: labor relations, contract negotiations, compensation, training and development, wage and salary administration, and career and personal counseling.

The aforementioned skills have been developed in both corporate and academic environments. Lois held senior management positions with municipal government as well as institutions of higher education including Rutgers University and Upsala College.

In 2000 Lois and her husband, Mitchell, entered the food business. Today, they own two McDonald's restaurants.

Lois is busy with community work and intercity youth. Presently, they employ over 200 intercity youth, mostly African Americans and Hispanics.

Lois has received many awards for her outstanding service to the community and is chairwoman of the Black McDonald's Owner/Operators Association Scholarship Fund, with $200,000 raised to date.

Lois, the mother of two children, is a native of New Jersey. She holds a BA in behavioral science and a MS in human resource management and counseling.

She and her husband have three grandchildren: twin girls, Ariana and Briana, age seven, and a grandson, Ryan, age two.

About the Four Contributors

Gary Smith

Gary W. Smith was raised in the small farming community of Bennett, Iowa. Upon graduating from high school, he went to college briefly. After discharge from the U.S. Navy, he worked in various machine shops as a journeyman, set-up man and foreman. He began a career at John Deere Harvester Works in 1979, retiring as a senior quality engineer and ISO 9000 management representative in 2007.

Gary's hobbies include doing home repairs and riding his Harley Davidson motorcycles. He is currently authoring a book on a new concept for Six Sigma Project methodology. Gary is a trustee at his United Methodist Church and truly believes that God's hand is at work in his life every day.

Gary was diagnosed with prostate cancer in July of 2009, just after his 57th birthday. He became friends with many at the University of Florida Proton Institute during his treatment protocol. Because of his experience with self-serving urologists after his diagnosis, and hearing the horror stories of his fellow patients, Gary has made it his goal to make all men aware that proton radiation is the best treatment available for low and medium Gleason score prostate cancers.

Bill Norrell

William (Bill) Norrell was born in 1942 in Chattanooga, Tennessee. The family moved to central Florida when he was in junior high school. He returned to Tennessee to care for his grandmother and he eventually completed his schooling there. After completing high school, he enlisted in the United States Army and served for three years.

After military service, Bill worked for a few companies to acquire some corporate experience. He began his lifetime career working for the United Sates Department of Agriculture and served as a federal/state supervisor, assistant regional director, and in various executive positions for 37 years.

His hobbies are golf, reading, and fishing. He also enjoys workouts in the gym with his wife, Vivian. They currently reside in Winter Haven, Florida.

Bill wanted to contribute to this book to help men understand that proton treatment for prostate cancer is a great option for maintaining quality of life. Although it is usually not even mentioned by urologists, it definitely turned out to be Bill's best option.

Paul Preuss

Paul Preuss was born in Brooklyn, New York, in 1942 and graduated from Richmond Hill High School in 1959. After graduating from Muhlenberg College, he left New York City behind and started his teaching career in Norwich, an upstate New York community of 10,000.

Paul married his college sweetheart, Becky, and she moved to Norwich where she began her teaching career as well. Paul and Becky lived in Norwich for 25 years, raising two sons while Paul earned degrees at Colgate and Syracuse University.

During this time, Paul entered school administration and served 21 years as a high school assistant principal and principal. In 1988, Paul left Norwich to become superintendent of schools in another school district.

He eventually moved on to become assistant superintendent at the regional Board of Cooperative Services (BOCES). This led him to greater contact with the New York State Education Department where he helped develop and advance a state-wide pilot system of Comprehensive District Education Planning (CDEP). This enabled Paul to retire earlier than planned and begin work as a private consultant and author on issues of root cause analysis and school improvement through the structured use of student data.

In earlier years Paul became a commercial hot air

balloon pilot and flew balloons as a hobby for 17 years. Other hobbies include photography, reading, boating, and travel. He loves "puttering" at his family retreat in Vermont.

In 2002 Paul and Becky moved to Queensbury, New York, near the shores of magnificent Lake George and less than two hours from their place in Vermont.

Paul was diagnosed with prostate cancer in August of 2009 and received his proton treatment during October, November, and December of that year at UFPTI. He is eager to share his experiences of treatment and follow-up with those who are facing similar decision-making issues.

Dan Cibock

Dan Cibock was born on January 31, 1955, in Chicago, Illinois. His family relocated to Rochester in 1968, a small town in northern Indiana. It was in this setting that Dan developed his love for nature and the great outdoors, which led to him pursuing a BS in biology from Indiana University in 1978.

One of many summer jobs Dan found during his college days was working for the Sonoco Products Plant in nearby Akron, Indiana. He continued to work at the plant after graduation, and joined the sales department in 1979. Over the years, he has relocated to five states and held several positions within the company. Dan is currently a customer service manager for the Industrial Carriers Division and lives in Florence, South Carolina. Dan has been an avid collector of brew paraphernalia for

40 years and loves to enjoy a good beer while cooking. His other hobbies include his yard, woodworking, and golf. Of course, in autumn, he becomes a loyal fan of Clemson and Chicago Bears football!

When Dan thinks of his experiences this past year with prostate cancer, all he can say is that he is so thankful to have known and worked with one particular gentleman the past 30 years. It was he who told Dan about a mutual friend who had undergone treatment in Jacksonville. It was through this individual that Dan found out about proton therapy and determined, after extensive research, that this was the form of treatment he wanted to pursue. Dan feels that he is so fortunate and all he can say is *Thank God!*

Patient Status
six months after treatment

Patient Name	PSA Before	PSA After	Side Effects	Duration
Bill Demboski	8.3	2.1	None	None
Mitch McGuire	5.8	1.6	Fatigue	3 Wks
Bill Norrell	2.1	0.80	Burning Urination Fatigue	2 Wks 2 Wks
Paul Preuss	5.0	2.1*	Freq.	Six Mo.
Gary Smith	5.4	1.6	None	None
Dan Cibock	4.70	2.1	Freq. of Urination	6-9 Mos.

*after three months

Comments by Patients:

Bill Demboski: I did not experience any post fatigue treatments. I resumed all my normal activities.

Paul Preuss: Frequency of urination remained higher than normal due to tightening of urethra resolved by Flomax. Hope to eventually wean myself off the drug in future.

Gary Smith: I had some urinary urgency during the last three weeks of treatments. I also experienced some fatigue during that time that lasted 3 weeks after treatment. No side effects were evident after 6 months. My 9 month PSA is 1.2 and dropping.

Mitchell McGuire returned home and found out his Dad was extremely ill and soon passed. He also had an elderly mother who was ill and he believes that combination caused depression, contributing to his fatigue. Mitchell has now recovered and is back to normal.

Contact Information

University of Florida Proton Therapy Institute
PH: 1-877-686-6009
Web site: Floridaproton.org

Bill Demboski	**bdemboski@comcast.net**
Karen Demboski	**bdemboski@comcast.net**
Mitchell McGuire	**capt4360@verizon.net**
Lois McGuire	**aka2341@verizon.net**
Gary Smith	**gary.smith.w@gmail.com**
Paul Preuss	**ppreuss@roadrunner.com**
Bill Norrell	**vnorrell@aol.com**
Dan Cibock	**bockdraft@yahoo.com**